Facing Death

Facing Death

Where Culture, Religion, and Medicine Meet

Edited by Howard M. Spiro, Mary G. McCrea Curnen, and Lee Palmer Wandel

*Prepared under the auspices of
The Program for Humanities in Medicine
Yale University School of Medicine
and
The Goethe-Institut, Boston*

Yale University Press   *New Haven and London*

Much of the material presented in Chapter 13 appeared in Valerie Hansen, 1995, *Negotiating Daily Life in Traditional China: How Ordinary People Used Contracts, 600–1400* (New Haven: Yale University Press).

Designed by Christopher Harris/Summer Hill Books.
Set in Galliard type by The Composing Room of Michigan, Inc., Grand Rapids, Michigan.
Printed in the United States of America by Edwards Brothers, Inc., Ann Arbor, Michigan.

Library of Congress Cataloging-in-Publication Data

Facing death / edited by Howard M. Spiro, Mary G. McCrea Curnen, Lee Palmer Wandel.
    p. cm.
    Prepared under the auspices of the Program for Humanities in Medicine, Yale University School of Medicine and the Goethe-Institut, Boston.
    Includes bibliographical references and index.
    ISBN 0-300-06349-0 (cloth : alk. paper)

    1. Terminally ill. 2. Death—Psychological aspects. 3. Death—Religious aspects.
4. Death—Moral and ethical aspects. I. Spiro, Howard M. (Howard Marget), 1924– .
II. Curnen, Mary G. McCrea. III. Wandel, Lee Palmer. IV. Yale University. Program for Humanities in Medicine. V. Goethe-Institut (Boston, Mass.)
R726.8.F33 1996
155.9'37—dc20   96-2487

A catalogue record for this book is available from the British Library.

The paper in this book meets the guidelines for permanence and durability of the Committee on Production Guidelines for Book Longevity of the Council on Library Resources.

10 9 8 7 6 5 4 3 2

To all those whose deaths have led us to meditate

Contents

Daniel Callahan

Ⅰt happens only once, and there is no chance to try again, to do it better the next time. What are we then to make of death—like birth, a once-in-a-lifetime event—and how might we best prepare for it? Of late there has been one widespread response to those questions: we should get ourselves a lawyer, or at least a form of some kind, and carefully specify how we want to die. A "death with dignity" is thought to be one marked by choice, by legal care, by giving thought to the medical treatment one does or does not want. If all of that is well in place, we are ready for death. So it is said.

Not quite. Put aside the fact that many of us will never get around to preparing advance directives, probably because we would rather think about something else. Anything else. Put aside also the fact that advance directives do not seem to make all that much difference in the way people are treated at the time of their death. Put aside the fact that only in America could one entertain the idea that a good preparation for death is to execute a legal document.

I do not mean here to deny the value or importance of advance directives. They may do some good, and I have duly prepared mine. I want instead only to note the oddity of the emphasis, the strange way in which a preparation for death is so often transposed from the personal to the legal, from the domain of self-reflection to that of pluralistic "choice," from the stuff of mystery, awe, and trepidation to that of medical and legal micromanagement. It is hard to think of a more clever way of avoiding the real subject altogether: the way we should understand death and situate it in our lives. We moderns no longer welcome a religious fix for such problems, but we seem quick to embrace a far less satisfying, even more evanescent, legal fix.

For all these reasons, a return to the more ancient tradition of *ars moriendi* is needed. Perhaps that tradition arose because earlier generations had to look death more directly in the face. Death was a daily companion that afflicted young and old, the weak and the strong, with almost equal ferocity. A walk in our old American cemeteries tells that story quite fully. Now we can hide death in hospitals and nursing homes, and we can hide it among the old, often well out of sight of the young. Perhaps too the tradition emerged because customs of self-examination, particularly the felt need to relate one's life and death to some larger scheme, flourished.

Whatever the reasons, it is time indeed to think once again about our dying and our death. AIDS has reminded us that the young do indeed die, and it cannot escape our notice that we ourselves will age and die—just as will or did our parents, grandparents, and everyone else before them.

But there is a difference between us and them. We are likely to die more slowly, over a long and uncertain period of time. Not for most of us will be the quick death from a virulent infection, now controlled by antibiotics, or even from a heart attack if the helicopter arrives in time. We will have to prepare ourselves for our death, watch it getting closer and closer, and wait for a moment that may take months or years to come—however surely we know it to be on the way. Our vigil is a blessing of modern medicine, even if at times it is its worst curse.

The tradition of *ars moriendi* understood one point of central importance: how we die will be a function of the way we have lived our lives and the kind of person we have become. I am reminded here of one of my favorite passages from the writing of Michel de Montaigne: "Fortune appears sometimes purposely to wait for the last years of our lives in order to show us she can overthrow in one moment what she has taken long years to build. In this last scene between ourselves and death, there is no more pretence. We must use plain words, and display such goodness or purity as we have at the bottom of the pot" (Montaigne 1958).

The papers collected in this volume will help us to reopen some old questions and to look differently at death. Death has been hidden of late under the weight of a technological medicine that would treat it as a kind of correctable accident, not a reality to be accepted as a fixed and necessary part of life. It has also been hidden by our modern unwillingness to talk much about how we ought to live our lives. In this way, death has become one more victim of what I have come to think of as the veil of pluralism, which forces the most intimate matters into the realm of the private and the personal—and thus puts them officially off limits for common reflection.

We have learned a great deal in our time about how lives may be saved and preserved, and a great deal about the causes and physiology of death. Now we need to learn once again how to go about our dying and what kind of a person that requires us to be. We need an *ars moriendi* no less than those who went to death long before us. If you think you know all about it already, you are lucky. I surely don't.

Reference

Montaigne, M. de. 1958. "That no man shall be called happy until after his death." In *The Essays of Montaigne,* trans. J. M. Cohen. New York: Penguin, 34–35.

Facing Death

Howard M. Spiro

Over the past century, technology has provided doctors and nurses with so much to keep death at bay that we have had very little time for contemplation or philosophy. As science turned mind into brain, it left no site at all for spirit. But now that social and economic forces have forced so much attention on the end of life, we as caregivers need to consider much more explicitly how people die. We must talk more about death itself, and we should talk in public. Among the many signs of reawakening interest are Sherwin Nuland's best-seller and Daniel Callahan's strictures on what should not be done. But few writers have specifically addressed the concerns of physicians and nurses, and that is what the editors hope this collection will do. For death, a forbidden topic too much for us, rarely makes it to Grand Rounds: our mortality conferences review why someone has died and what errors may have been made, but we never wonder aloud whether it could have been the right time for that patient to die. We talk in euphemisms of euthanasia, but leave it to a literary figure to talk, however ironically, of "a very good death."

Once, when grandparents, parents, and sometimes children—too often children—died at home, everyone knew death first hand. Death is as common as birth, but it went into hiding in our twentieth-century hospitals. Foreigners may have made fun of the American banishment of death—and did—but Europe was little better, for even there death had replaced sex as the forbidden subject, as several of our contributors point out.

Sometimes death comes a little earlier or a little later. But warnings by the Puritan divines of New England that we are all in the hands of an angry God who at any moment might let us fall into the fiery furnace get very little attention from their descendants. Death is no longer destiny, but the failure of doctors, written nowhere in God's plan. Death can be repelled, repulsed almost forever—a disease that doctors should be able to cure.

AIDS AND VIOLENCE

Today the twin epidemics of AIDS and violence, which kill so many young people, have forced the attention of almost everyone back on death at a time when resources consumed and money spent have made economists and government officials also worry about how long it takes for the elderly to die in our hospitals. Television shows us how shootings and trauma rip at life and make our inner cities seem like battlefields. Fatalism has gained new strength from the mayhem in the streets and from the early death of those with AIDS as the prospect of early death makes risk-taking easy and the pursuit of pleasures more alluring. *Carpe diem* was the way it once was phrased. AIDS too has its own battlefield, its obituaries easy to decode: anyone dying under age forty is likely to have died of AIDS, or a gunshot; only in those over age sixty can one confidently expect death from some other reason. But even if death from AIDS turns public, life with AIDS remains too private. AIDS may have been transformed from a crisis that once filled doctors with dread into an everyday event, but its stigma persists.

REBIRTH OF DEATH

To tell the truth, death is doing very well these days. Dr. Kevorkian, whose obligatory honorific underlines the oxymoron of "doctor" and "death," has made euthanasia as acceptable for table talk as managed health care. One might hope that interest has grown because physicians and nurses, like the public, are becoming more philosophical; but issues of scarcity, rationing, and overspending are more plausible stimuli. Medical care, optimistically renamed "health care," is now talked of as an industry where death represents a product like any other in our modern hospitals. Dying takes so much time and has so many variations that its costs are unpredictable, often outlandish, and destructive of the "bottom line." Families and even doctors and nurses may grieve at the prolonged futility that extends dying, but it is the growing cost that brings the most dismay. The unwelcome guest at the feast of technology is death done up as rationing.

DYING IN THE HOSPITAL

In big hospital wards during the first half of this century, with thirty patients in two rows, dying was no stranger; drawn curtains told the silent story. Only when the big wards were replaced by small rooms did death disappear, for a while, behind closed doors. In our Western world most people are born into technology and leave it only when they die. The comfortable deaths of fiction, the ways of dying—*ars moriendi*—have been replaced by the battle in the hospital. Now once again patients die more visibly, in intensive-care-unit cubicles where doctors and nurses pound on their chests and shout instructions as they scan the video monitors. Relatives can only watch behind a tangle of life-supporting, death-delaying apparatus. Goethe could never have asked for more light in an intensive care unit, and would not have needed to, so bright are the lights already.

Few can turn quietly to the wall to go peacefully. For one thing, hospitals are too expensive a place to await a quiet death. For another, we doctors and nurses are not good at waiting. Our house staff are young and confident, eager to prove their mettle. In intensive care units the dying find no rest, but are kept in motion by machines blowing up their lungs and beating their hearts; electrical connections sometimes seem more important than the bodies they serve. There are few last words from dying patients because most have tubes in their throats; the staff are too busy shouting orders to hear them anyway. There hardly seems room in these crowded cubicles for the rest that the Angel of Death brings. The image of Prometheus, the eagle gnawing at his eternal liver, might serve as a more fitting emblem.

Prolonged dying is what has united us all, not death itself. That is why people sign wills and durable powers of attorney with instructions about the ways in which they want to be kept alive or die. How we die worries us the most, because, despite all the legal harness, that remains almost beyond our control. Doctors debate the technology of prolonged dying, but we talk little about the philosophical, cultural, symbolic, or welcome aspects of death—some think because physicians fear death more than do many others.

In the reductionist world of physicians and nurses, death has become a purely physical process: when someone has died is no longer a matter for lay people to decide; instead it has become a highly technical and sometimes contentious judgment. The Creator may have breathed life into Adam, but breath no longer defines the living, and putting a mirror to the nostrils to determine whether someone still lives seems naive. For a while, electrocardiograms served to show when the heart stopped, until pacemakers came along to keep the heart beating almost forever. Electroencephalograms, the next guide, generated arguments over how few brain waves meant "brain death," or about how much and which part of the brain could go before the body could be called dead. Organs are "harvested" from those who are "brain dead," and many now live thanks to those livers, kidneys, lungs, and hearts. But are they donors or gardens? Shall we call donors corpses if they can still breathe with a machine? Does the soul depend on a respirator? Is the soul released only when the plug is pulled? The questions seem endless, and yet we doctors only praise the benefits. I sometimes think that the transplantation of organs is like a sacrament and that it deserves a certificate, an attestation, to the rite of passage that it represents.

The spiritual aspects of death are almost entirely ignored in medical training. During the clinical years of medical school when textbooks are studied most, philosophical and religious considerations get little formal attention. Premedical students must take four or five courses in science and mathematics, but none are required in history, anthropology, religion, or philosophy. They do not get any training from which they may learn how different people have dealt with death—or life. Further, the work of doctors and nurses ends with the death of the patient. Few of us go to patients' funerals, and we rarely reflect on the nature of the world in which we live. We forget because our duties at hospital and office seem so different from our lives at home.

For a while, the clergy mostly let the bandwagon for death roll by. Familiar figures in the hospitals of the 1940s and 1950s before resuscitation made visiting so difficult, by the late 1950s and 1960s they had become rare visitors to our wards except as psychotherapists. Since the 1990s, however, the clergy have returned, and conversations with them will grow increasingly helpful to doctors and nurses if we all are careful to respect our different perspectives. Physicians, doubters as well as believers, have to be careful in how we attempt to explain away religious experience. We need to talk more with philosophers, historians, and the clergy to remember that men and women are more than the bodies we repair, and that dying comes to all. Culture and tradition—and religion—help doctors and nurses, as well as our patients, at times of crisis. All of the editors hope that this book will serve as a starting point for that conversation.

A GOOD DEATH AT HOME

People rarely get a chance to die at home with family and friends. Strangers taking care of strangers, physicians, nurses, and other hospital personnel know mostly the bodies smashed in an accident, broken by bullets, silent after a stroke, or in shock from the breakdown of an internal organ. Our job is to sew up the wound or repair what has fallen apart, right what is wrong, and let the unknown details sort themselves out later. Only hospice has come along to share our burden, to make dying more comfortable and more visible as part, once again, of the community of the living.

A "good death" is a death at home, but it requires family being available and a dying that is not prolonged. In hospitals, personal relationships are replaced by interactions with the team that shares the medical duties with the physician and nurse. The technology that prolongs life presses the same way of dying on us all; religion, character, accomplishment, all the links to the past are lost in the uniformity of hospital death. Somewhere Rilke cried, "O Lord, give everyone his own death."

Patients don't just die in medical parlance; they often "die on us," a phrase that suggests that someone else must be to blame. Physicians rarely see death, in Lee Wandel's felicitous phrase, as defining part of life. Rather for us it is the enemy, the defeat of all that we do. We never praise death.

The death of the young has become common and the death of the aged has become prolonged by "life support" systems in the web of "managed care" and "risk management." We will look for no final answers, but only for some of the right questions.

A PERSONAL NOTE

It may not be fair to blame this century's inattention to death only on doctors and nurses. Numbness—"alexithymia," one psychiatrist called it— may have replaced pain as the complaint of our century now that aspirin analgesia, nonsteroidal anti-inflammatory agents (NSAIDs), and other an-odynes can take away the pains of the civilized world. But to the earth-quakes and floods, to all our world's catastrophes in their ancient rhythms, the twentieth century has added the death camps of Europe, and the massa-cres in Africa, Asia, and—once again—in Europe.

And yet, strolling through the campus as I do on my way to and from work on pleasant days, especially in spring, I find myself gazing at the grand buildings of its college. I gain inspiration from the way they are transformed with the changing light of the seasons. The faces have changed in my four decades here and I rejoice in these changes. The hereafter may be only a metaphor, and the Creator only our hope, but the immortality of the human race surely is manifest in the students who will become the citizens and teachers of tomorrow.

My generation has lived through so much, has witnessed so many sor-rows, and we doctors have always known grief. Yet I remain full of hope, joyful for the future, maybe because I have worked in a university all of my adult life. . . .

ARS MORIENDI

On April 15–16, 1994, a colloquium on *ars moriendi,* not so much the art of dying as the *way* of dying, took place at Yale University School of Medicine in New Haven, Connecticut. Jointly sponsored by the Program for Humanities in Medicine at Yale and by the Goethe-Institut, Boston, it was a conference in which, first, medical caregivers told of their own reactions to death. Next, philosophers, historians, and the clergy related how some cultures have dealt with death and how religious experience has shaped it. Finally, the modern plague of AIDS was remembered by participants looking for a deeper understanding of the emotional and spiritual needs of the dying—as well as for those who care for them.

The conference, like this book derived from it, had several parts; but here we have gathered those parts into two sections—Witnessing Death: The Medical Battle, and Framing Death: Cultural and Religious Responses. The sudden deaths of trauma and violence, the gunshot deaths that should arouse our anger, we pass by here, for those deaths deserve far fuller consideration than our pages allow. The conference made clear that we in the caring professions do not need as much to be reacquainted with death as to stop ignoring it. We doctors and nurses have simply to open our eyes to what we do—and our hearts and minds to what we fear. We need to contemplate, and talk about, death. We need once again to express our grief when our patients die and our anger that defeat sometimes brings. We need to feel.

Note

I dedicate this preface to the memory of Enid Peschel, cofounder and codirector of the Program for Humanities in Medicine at Yale who died suddenly on August 15, 1994, before fulfilling her mission of convincing others that mental illness is brain disease. We all miss Enid every day.

The editors have many to thank. The most important is Professor Arthur Imhof of the Free University of Berlin. Professor Imhof came to Yale in the spring of 1992 to give us his thoughts on the "art of dying." A demographer and historian, he brought us a new understanding of what it was that had happened to the rituals of death. Together we conceived of a conference focusing on the dilemmas of the people who take care of the dying: physicians, nurses, and other medical care workers—or as they have come to be known, health care professionals. It was Professor Imhof's inspiration, his many years of preparation, that made this conference possible.

Dr. Peter Schmitt, Director of the Goethe-Institut in Boston, Massachusetts, was our helper and collaborator from the very beginning. It was he who brought Professor Imhof to us, and it was he who supplied the energy and some of the finances to make our program possible. We are grateful to him as well as to Kathryn Conti, Program Coordinator of the Goethe-Institut, Boston. These helpful collaborations make our world a better place.

Eva Schuster of the Art Museum in Düsseldorf was kind enough to join us with an exhibit of photographs from her memorable collection, now fortunately in book form, though not yet in English. (*Das Bild Vom Tod*, 1992). We regret that we could not supply the reader with a full representation of her collection.

There are many others to thank. Dr. James Kenney and Janice Gore ensured the success of our meeting with their organizational skills. Clara Gyorgyey, Priscilla and Will Norton, and Tamma McNeil all contributed in their various ways. Patricia Perona helped enormously in the preparation of the final manuscripts. We should not forget the students and other participants in the program as well as the audience, whose many good questions, sadly, could not be reprinted here. We express our gratitude for their stimulating thoughts.

We all wish to thank Mary G. McCrea Curnen for her organizational and managerial skills, which inspired a large number of authors to submit their contributions on time. Our thanks also goes to Jean Thomson Black, science editor at Yale University Press, and to her colleagues at the press who helped us in so many ways. We are most grateful to Ethel Symolon, cataloguing assistant at the Yale Center for British Art, who assisted us in selecting the illustration for the cover of this book.

Defining a Life: The Western Tradition

Lee Palmer Wandel

In the two decades after 1300, an exiled Florentine civil servant wrote a poem of one hundred cantos in which he, in the middle of his life, "nel mezzo del cammin di nostra vita," encountered thousands of people both long and recently dead. Historians usually write of the dead, but I know of no other work of literature whose population is predominantly, let alone almost exclusively, the souls of dead men and women. That poem is Dante Alighieri's *Comedia,* or *Divine Comedy* as it came to be called.[1] That poem is appropriate to open a volume on death and dying, not because it is about dead people, but because each of the dead whom Dante meets during his pilgrimage is located purposefully and precisely on the maps of Hell, Purgatory, or Paradise that he has drawn for us in words. Each person's location in death was determined by his or her life—what sort of life each had lived.

THE BIOLOGICAL MODEL OF HUMANITY

I draw upon Dante's magnificent and powerful poem to wrench us out of our contemporary sensibilities, which are so dominated by biology—to wrench us out of this time when we accept tacitly, if not expressly, the conception of human beings as organisms. This view is articulated most frequently within the medical community, but it is pervasive in many public debates. In our discussions of assisted death, we increasingly accept physical suffering as a justification, though we have not yet reached consensus as to the threshold of that suffering. But what of the loss of dignity inflicted by intestinal cancer, chronicled so thoughtfully in Sherwin Nuland's *How We Die?* What of the loss of both dignity and the very person him- or herself—the wit, the personality, the individual charms and strengths of character, the humor, the foibles—that Alzheimer's and other diseases of the brain work upon human beings? These losses do not constitute suffering of the same kind or weight, according to that biological model. So, too, this conception of human beings as organisms frames both sides of the abortion debate: women are "bodies," fetuses are "alive," and those two inadequate statements delimit the discussion. It undercuts the efforts of so many different kinds of people whose motor skills, visual agility, patterns of thought, or modes of speaking differ from the normative organism, to live in the world and not away from it. Finally, that conception has come to dominate how we think of the days, weeks, months, and even years in people's lives that follow the diagnosis of certain kinds of illness: "terminal illness," with its certain prognosis of death. Thus it is that my friend was told she was "terminal" some eight months before she died. Thus it is that we speak of people dying of AIDS and cancer, not living. Dante serves to underline the vacuity of that language: Toward what end?

ANOTHER WORLD, ANOTHER WAY OF THINKING ABOUT HUMANITY

> Le but de nostre carrière, c'est la mort,
> c'est l'object necessaire de nostre visée.
> [The goal of our career is death. It is the
> necessary object of our aim.]
> —Montaigne, *Essais*

Let me return you for a while to a different time, when suffering and death were constants, and how one lived was the variable. That time is not so distant: aspirin, ether, penicillin, and other antibiotics are modern inventions. Not until around 1900 could doctors alleviate the pain of arthritis, rheumatism, migraines, and other forms of minor, yet chronic, physical pain. Not until the 1930s were penicillin and other antibiotics applied to stop virulent and often fatal bacterial infections such as tuberculosis, bacterial pneumonia, venereal diseases, and a variety of postoperative infections (for example, septicemia and staphylococci). Until the mid-nineteenth century, the prevalent painkillers were alcohol and death itself: the people of the past lived with toothaches, migraines, sinus infections and headaches, arthritis, rheumatism, and the pain of cancer. They knew all illnesses and accidents as potentially fatal; as Montaigne observed, a simple bump above the ear from a tennis ball could be deadly. They knew, as we seem to have forgotten, that death comes, usually unexpectedly, to everyone. Life was not defined by pain; pain was a constant in the lives of the "healthy" as well as the ill. Nor was life defined by death; *every* life had its terminus in death. Life was not organic, a chemical process that might be interrupted at any point by other organisms—it was defined by how one lived. As Montaigne speculated, all life was a preparation for death. He did not mean that life was to be lived in death's shadow, but rather, as Dante made so palpable, that the consequences of how one lived were eternal.

That conception unites the period in which I wish to dwell for a bit, and divides it from the modern world. In some form, it was held by a wide range of different cultures, religions, and traditions: Greek and Roman, medieval, early modern, early American (even, to a certain degree, nineteenth century); Judaism, Western and Eastern Christianity, and Islam; classical, Christian, even Enlightenment and Revolutionary. This essay cannot pretend to offer a comprehensive overview or even a representative summary of all the different formulations that conception received as it was articulated in these different cultures, religions, and traditions. It does not offer here perspectives from non-European traditions, nor from Judaism or Islam, many of which others will address. Rather, I offer from my own training, my own reading, a handful of views that meditate on what it is to be human. Each author takes up the dichotomy, body/soul, at the center of the Western tradition. Each explores the relation of the body to the soul. For each, that relation is different, from complete severability to complete interdependence, because each conceives differently both what a body is—what it means for humans to "have bodies"—and what the soul is. Each explores the relation of mental functions such as reason and imagination to something more elusive, something not the same as reason or emotion, something we call the "soul," in Greek, *psyche,* in Latin, *animus.* For all, that "soul" was what distinguished human beings from the rest of the natural world or creation. For all, each human being had a soul, and that soul was unique to that person, different from every other soul. One's soul is that which distinguishes one from every other person; thereafter, differences of kin, citizenship, or nationality might matter. One's soul gives direction, either good or bad, to one's life. For four authors, each person's soul is immortal.

The works treated here are all European,[2] and their authors range from a fifth-century B.C. Athenian to three Christians to one probable atheist. They have in common that they all had an impact on how others formulated the question of human nature and conceived of the relation between the physical and the spiritual in human beings. Each shaped subsequent debates by defining elementary terms and framing the questions that others would pursue. All of these works have a resilience: each reading provokes new thoughts, enriches one's perspective. I offer them here because, as a historian, I believe we still have much to learn from the past. At the least, we can be reminded that we do not need to think of things in the ways we do; at best, we can rediscover other perspectives that enable us to enrich, enlarge, even shift our own.

A GREEK VIEW

One of the earliest Europeans to address the question of the soul, both its relation to the body and its immortality, was Socrates, who was first made famous by his pupil Plato. In 399 B.C., Socrates was accused by three other citizens, brought to trial, allowed to speak in his own defense, found guilty of corrupting the young and believing in gods other than those officially recognized in Athens, allowed to plead for the form of punishment he wished, and then condemned to die by poison. The fullest account of those last days is to be found in four dialogues Plato wrote. The line separating Plato's craft from Socrates' speaking is difficult, perhaps impossible to discern. In Plato's dialogues, his beloved teacher articulates what he believes his life was about:

> Perhaps someone may say, 'But surely, Socrates, after you have left us you can spend the rest of your life in quietly minding your own business.' This is the hardest thing of all to make some of you understand. If I say that this would be disobedience to God, and that is why I cannot 'mind my own business,' you will not believe that I am serious. If, on the other hand, I tell you that to let no day pass without discussing goodness and all the other subjects about which you hear me talking and examining both myself and others is really the very best thing that a man can do, and that life without this sort of examination is not worth living, you will be even less inclined to believe me. Nevertheless that is how it is, gentlemen (Plato 1954, 71–72).

Socrates believed that life could not be lived in isolation. For Socrates as Plato presented him, the truly good life was lived in dialectic with other human beings in pursuit of understanding. The purpose of life was the education of the soul in what at least Plato called "the Good." Socrates' life was defined by the dialogues he pursued, the "examination" he conducted, his exchanges with others in the pursuit of understanding of the Good. In those dialogues, we watch Socrates provoke with his "rough words" the Athenian jury first to find him guilty, and then to condemn him to death. Why?[3] As Socrates explained to his grieving friends in the *Phaedo*, he was seventy; soon his body would begin to decay, as did everything physical, and it would impede the progress of his soul toward true knowledge. Socrates did not fear death, but rather the loss of that which had defined his life—his pursuit of the knowledge of "the Good." That loss could take place in two ways: he could be banned from speaking, ordered to stop that dialectical examination of the nature of the Good; or the infirmities of old age could weaken him so much that he could no longer pursue the Good.

Socrates did not fear death because, as he argued in Plato's *Phaedo,* the immortality of the soul was incontrovertible. The body decayed and died; but the soul was immortal. For Plato, and possibly for Socrates, that soul had three aspects or parts. As Plato described in *The Republic,* these parts were the intellectual; the "spiritual," in the sense that horses have "spirit"; and the animal, or physical. Each person was dominated by one of these aspects of the soul: philosophers by the intellectual, soldiers by the spiritual, and manual laborers and hedonists by the third. Each was distinguished by a particular balance among those three aspects; only in philosopher-kings were the three in perfect balance. At the end of the *Republic,* Plato posed his vision of the immortality of the soul, which would return again and again to the new bodies of human infants to continue its education in the Good. As long as souls resided in bodies, that education would never be perfect.

A CHRISTIAN OF THE LATE ROMAN EMPIRE: AUGUSTINE

Socrates' conviction redefines death not as the terminus, but as a doorway. It reorients. That reorientation has never been more eloquently chronicled than in Augustine's great prayer to God, the *Confessio,* or *Confession.* There Augustine articulates the process by which he was turned from that "life" one lives in the body—from the pleasures of eating, of sexual play, of beautiful speaking, rhetoric, of writing, poetry, and of sound, music—to see in the life of the body "death," and in death the "life" of the soul. The *Confession* describes Augustine's private and personal *conversio*—his reorientation from the world defined by the experiences and pleasures of the body, to the world defined by the yearning of the soul for its source and telos, God. To translate into terms that would have resonance for the next millennium, it was a reorientation from "this world" to the "other world." For Augustine, the presence of the soul within each human being was the clearest evidence of God—an imperfect, partially clouded perception of immortality. The soul offered the merest glimpse of eternity, omnipotence, of infinite Goodness—Plato's Good transformed into the Christian God.

The *Confession* is a chronicle of one soul's reorientation. At the end of his life, as his home, Hippo, faced obliteration by the Visigoths, Augustine worked out most fully the implications of that reorientation in *The City of God (Civitas dei).* There he described two cities "created by two kinds of

love: the earthly city was created by self-love reaching the point of contempt for God, the Heavenly City by the love of God carried as far as
contempt of self" (Augustine 1984, 593). Those two cities did not corre-
spond to Rome and Heaven, but to two human communities: those who
were oriented to "this world" as it would come to be designated, the world
"of the body"—the world of physical pleasure and pain—and those oriented toward the "other world," the world the soul inhabits in its quest for
God. For Augustine, that reorientation embraced all human history, every
human being—those long dead, those alive, those yet to be born. All
belonged to one city or the other.

Like Plato, Augustine held that the soul was immortal. Augustine conceived of that immortality differently, however. It was not a long, perhaps
infinite series of returns to bodies in a process of education. The soul, for
Augustine, belonged to only one body, which died, and whose final resurrection Augustine addressed in *The City of God*. At death, the soul "crossed
over" from "this world" to the "other." Those who had lived in anticipation
of the other world would ultimately join God on the Day of the Last
Judgment—those whose souls had yearned for fulfillment in the divinity
would be fulfilled beyond all imagining. And those who had lived in "this
world," the world of the body, were condemned to an eternity of unhappiness, for they could never be fulfilled. In Augustine, in other words, we
find the reorientation of human life: only a negligible portion of it was
lived in "this world"; immortality of the soul, within the Christian tradition, meant an eternity *after* death. One's biological life was spent in preparation for and anticipation of that eternal "life," or it was not. The choice
lay with each human being, and each soul had its own inner compass
toward the world of the "flesh," the body, or toward God. Each choice had
consequences for eternity, because God, argued Augustine, could not be
reached through the world of the flesh.

For more than a millennium following Augustine, Christians would look
forward to death as the portal through which they might enter the heaven
that Dante would seek to describe; to "live," following the late antique
translation of the two notions "life" and "death," eternally after they had
died. Montaigne records the story of Saint Hilary, who prayed for the early
death of his daughter, that she might thereby remain innocent and pure,
rather than marry and become more "physical," bound to the world of the
body, of sexual relations and childbearing: "His design was to make her
lose the desire and habit of worldly pleasures in order to unite her wholly
to God; but as the shortest and surest means to this end seemed to him to
be the death of his daughter, he did not cease, by vows, prayers, and

orisons, to request God to take her from this world and call her to himself."
Hilary was blessed and his daughter died. Hilary's wife, upon hearing of his
achievement with God, asked that he do the same for her, and so he prayed.
Soon thereafter, she died: "Hers was a death embraced with singular unani-
mous contentment" (Montaigne 1957, 162; 1965, 219). Life, for that millennium, did not reside in the body, but with God.

Christians, however, as Augustine warned them, were forbidden to has-
ten that death through suicide. The vision of the divine ordering of the
universe that Augustine and then Dante sought to articulate meant that
every human being had a place in sacred history and that no human being
could know *before* death what that place was—the meaning of each human
life was hidden until the final day. Human beings could, following orthodox theology, participate in the formation of their lives, the definition of
their lives, and to them fell the responsibility for what kind of eternal "life"
each would live. But God alone determined the place and time of death,
when and where one could enter the portal, when and where the life of
"this world" ended and the life of the "other" began.

A MEDIEVAL CHRISTIAN: DANTE

Augustine divided human lives according to the orientation of each
person's love: the self, or those who inhabited the earthly city, and God, or
those who inhabited the Heavenly City. For Dante, too, what defined a life
was love:

> "Nè creator nè creatura mai,"
>   cominciò el "figliuol, fu sanza amore,
>   o naturale o d'animo; e tu 'l sai.
> Lo naturale è sempre sanza errore,
>   ma l'altro puote errar per malo obietto
>   o per troppo o per poco di vigore."

["Neither Creator nor creature, my son, was ever without love, either natural or
of the mind," he began, "and this thou knowest; the natural is always without
error, but the other may err through a wrong object or through excess or defect
of vigour."]

"Purgatorio," canto 17[4]

Human lives were divided not only according to the object of their love,
but also according to the strength of that love. Dante, moreover, distinguished among the objects of love. For him, there were more than two foci,

self or God. There were many kinds of human and divine love. In Hell, excessive love of the physical began with other persons, Paolo and Francesca, near the entrance to Hell; descended through gluttony, avarice, and love of self; and culminated in the complete absence of love, treachery. In Purgatory, imperfect forms of love mirrored the tiers of Hell, moving from love whose objects were themselves inappropriate, such as pride and envy ("love perverted," in the words of John Sinclair); through weak love; to excessive love, which ranged from attachments of the body to pleasures and wealth; to that excessive love of others Christians called lust. In Paradise, love ascended in ever greater forms of perfection, culminating in Saint Bernard's chaste prayer to the Virgin and Dante's own beatific vision.

> All'alta fantasia qui mancò possa;
> ma già volgeva il mio disio e 'l velle,
> sì come rota ch' igualmente è mossa,
> l'amor che move il sole e l'altre stelle.

[Here power failed the high phantasy; but now my desire and will, like a wheel that spins with even motion, were revolved by the Love that moves the sun and the other stars.]

"Paradiso," canto 33

For Dante, the soul was drawn to God in love; love moved the will to choose some objects over others. Love was the name he gave to that which moved the sun and the other stars and moved the soul to aspire to God. That love, for Dante, still divided between the "flesh"—the vices of lust, avarice, and gluttony in Hell and Purgatory—and "the spirit." But spiritual love, as one found in Paradise, might be directed to human beings. The theologians would name that love *caritas;* for Aquinas and others, it had its origin and its telos in God, but it found expression in "this world" toward one's neighbor. For Dante, all souls, but perhaps three, loved. It was their choice of object, the telos of that love, that divided souls. It was possible, he suggested through the stories in the "Paradiso," to love God in the world. And the *Divine Comedy,* with its verbal invocations of places, sensations, colors, sounds, smells, even textures—its location of the reader in the darkness, the stenches, the geography, the muck of Hell or the brilliant, mystical rose of Paradise—is among the most physically intricate acts of worship of a soul in search of God.

The *Divine Comedy* offers us a glimpse of medieval sensibilities toward the dead: the living Dante walks among the spirits of thousands of dead men and women, talking with them, learning their individual stories, discerning their individual destinies. Perhaps nowhere can we *see* so explicitly the implications of Christian anthropology. By the fourteenth century, many Europeans were living comfortably with the dead. The bones of saints, relics, formed foci of worship, places where the devout felt closer to God—here Christians could touch the physical remains of those who had lived more fully in the "other" world. So, too, families prayed to their own dead kin, who they hoped were "living next to God," whose immortal souls resided on the right side of God the Father and who they hoped might "speak" to God on behalf of their relatives still living in the world of the body. Until the modern day, European Christians believed the souls of the dead could hear the requests and the prayers of the living—death did not sever them completely from those still in "this world." As the Reformers would decry in the sixteenth century, the dead dominated the living, receiving not only their prayers, but also their wealth, in the form of endowed masses and indulgences, those petitions of clemency to the Pope. The Christian conception of the immortality of the soul had made the world a rather crowded place.

A RENAISSANCE CHRISTIAN: MONTAIGNE

The sixteenth-century essayist, diplomat, and humanist Michel de Montaigne posed a different understanding of the soul and its relation to the body. In his essay the *Apology for Raymond Sebond* he took up the linkage that Christian scholars from Augustine through Luther had maintained between the soul and the mind: that the mind was the location for pure analytic reasoning, that it could function autonomously of the body, and that it was linked to the soul, which Christian theology had maintained could be separated from the body (Montaigne 1957, 318–457; 1965, 436–604). Indeed, Plato would argue that pure reasoning was possible only in the mind that had become as independent as possible from the body. In the *Apology,* Montaigne asked his famous question, ¿*Que sçay-je?* (What do I know?) In answering, he repudiated the claim of natural theology that man could know God through the application of his reason to the natural world. Montaigne placed the mind fully in the body. The mind received all of its information through those same senses Plato had decried as distorting. It was susceptible to all the emotions, which had their seat in the body, vulnerable to the fluctuations of sensation the body experienced, subject to sensations that confused or disoriented. Its only media of expression were physical, corporal: speaking was sounds, gestures were bodily movements, and writing required both the hand and the eye. The mind, in other words, belonged to the world of the body. It "knew," in the sense that Plato, Augustine, and even Dante would mean, nothing:

> Finalement, il n'y a aucune constante existence, ny de nostre estre, ny de celuy des objects. Et nous, et nostre jugement, et toutes choses mortelles, vont coulant et roulant sans cesse. Ainsin il ne se peut establir rien de certain de l'un à l'autre, et le jugeant et le jugé estans en continuelle mutation et branle (Montaigne 1965, 601).

> [Finally, there is no existence that is constant, either of our being or of that of objects. And we, and our judgment, and all mortal things go on flowing and rolling unceasingly. Thus nothing certain can be established about one thing by another, both the judging and the judged being in continual change and motion] (Montaigne 1957, 455).

What of the soul? Montaigne's concern in the *Apology* was to sever human intellectual activity such as Socrates had pursued from faith in God's existence. The soul was the location of faith. That faith assured one of the certain existence of God, but that certainty was not the product of human intellection nor of human physical experience. The certainty of faith differed in essence both from the knowledge the mind acquired and from the knowledge experience brought. These latter two forms of knowledge were interdependent and both were flawed. The certainty of the soul came unmediated from God:

> Ny que l'homme se monte au dessus de soy et de l'humanité: car il ne peut voir que de ses yeux, ny saisir que de ses prises. Il s'eslevera si Dieu lui preste extraordinairement la main; il s'eslevera, abandonnant et renonçant à ses propres moyens, et se laissant hausser et soubslever par la grâce divine: mais non autrement (Montaigne 1965, 604).

> [Nor can man raise himself above himself and humanity; for he can see only with his own eyes, and seize only with his own grasp. He will rise, if God lends him his hand; he will rise by abandoning and renouncing his own means, and letting himself be raised and uplifted by divine grace; but not otherwise] (Montaigne 1957, 457, n. 66).

Montaigne did not repudiate the body. Quite the contrary, to be human, for Montaigne, was to live in a body of particular senses, to think, finally, somatically. To be human was to *be* a body. It was also, however, to have a soul, that place where man and God were connected and into which grace came. The body was the source and the seat of human knowledge; the soul was the recipient of knowledge of God. In an age of religious wars, Mon-

taigne argued for a different understanding both of the body, as that fluctu-
ating medium through which all human beings acquired whatever knowledge they claimed, and of the soul, still immortal, but more cleanly and
immediately touched by God.

THE FRENCH ENLIGHTENMENT PHILOSOPHE: DIDEROT

Sometime in the 1760s, Denis Diderot, the philosophe and author of the
great publishing venture of the Enlightenment, the *Encyclopedia,* began
writing the short dialogue *Rameau's Nephew.* He did not publish it in his
own lifetime; it would appear first in German, in Goethe's translation, in
1805. In it, Diderot explored the most radical implications of Montaigne's
speculations: the possibility that human beings have no constant nature at
all. He posed a man of constantly changing manner, appearance, and even
voice:

> Rien ne dissemble plus de lui que lui-même. Quelquefois, il est maigre et hâve,
> comme un malade au dernier degré de la consomption; on compterait ses dents à
> travers ses joues. On dirait qu'il a passé plusiers jours sans manger, ou qu'il sort
> de la Trappe. Les mois suivant, il est gras et replet, comme s'il n'avait pas quitté la
> table d'un financier, ou qu'il eût été renfermé dans un couvent de Bernardins
> (Diderot 1972, 32).

> [He has no greater opposite than himself. Sometimes he is thin and wan like a
> patient in the last stages of consumption; you could count his teeth through his
> skin; he looks as if he had been days without food or had just come out of a
> Trappist monastery. The next month, he is sleek and fat as if he ate regularly at a
> banker's or had shut himself up in a Bernardine convent] (Diderot 1956, 9).

He is a consummate actor, capable of any role, any "position," as he called
it—able to play buffoon, his favorite, or brilliant musician, to mimic ge-
nius. The only constants in his life are hunger, thirst, and sexual needs:

> MOI. . . . Qu'avez-vous fait?
> LUI. Ce que vous, moi et tous les autres font; du bien, du mal et rien. Et puis j'ai
> eu faim, et j'ai mangé, quand l'occasion s'en est présentée; après avoir mangé, j'ai
> eu soif, et j'ai bu quelquefois. Cependant la barbe me venait; et quand elle a été
> venue, je l'ai fait raser.
> MOI. Vous avez mal fait. C'est la seule chose qui vous manque, pour être un sage
> (Diderot 1972, 35).

> [MYSELF. . . . What have you been doing?

HE. What you and I and the rest do, namely good and evil, and also nothing. And then I was hungry and I ate when I had the chance. After eating I was thirsty and I have occasionally drunk. Meanwhile my beard grew and when grown I had it shaved.
MYSELF. There you did wrong. A beard is all you lack to be a sage] (Diderot 1956, 11).

In Rameau's nephew, Diderot has drawn a "natural man," a parody of his near contemporary, Rousseau. Here is someone whose "nature" is not merely in "flux," as Montaigne had posed. What defines him are the demands of "his bowels," and the roles he is willing to play to satiate those demands. He is the antithesis of Socrates' conception of human nature:

> LUI. . . . Voilà où vous en êtes, vous autres. Vous croyez que le même bonheur est fait pour tous. Quelle étrange vision! Le vôtre suppose une certain tour d'espirit romanesque que nous n'avons pas; une âme singulière, un goût particulier. Vous décorez cette bizarrerie du nom de vertu; vous l'appelez philosophie. Mais la vertu, la philosophie sont'elles fait pour tout le monde. . . . Tenez, vive la philosophie; vive la sagesse de Salomon: Boire de bon vin, se gorger de mets délicats; se rouler sur de jolies femmes; se reposer dans des lits bien mollets. Excepté cela, le reste n'est que vanité (Diderot 1972, 65).

> [HE. . . . That's where you fellows are behind the times. You think everybody aims at the same happiness. What an idea! Your conception presupposes a sentimental turn of mind which is not ours, an unusual spirit, a special taste. You call your quirks virtue, or philosophy. But virtue and philosophy are not made for everybody. . . . Listen! I say hurrah for wisdom and philosophy— the wisdom of Solomon: to drink good wines, gorge on choice food, tumble pretty women, sleep in downy beds—outside of that, all is vanity] (Diderot 1956, 34–35).

In *Rameau's Nephew,* Diderot proposes the possibility that for some human beings, at least, there might be nothing more to them than the roles they played; their "nature" is essentially imitative, mimicking the gestures, the behavior, even the beliefs of others. Not unlike Augustine's citizens of the City of Man, Rameau's nephew seems to live simply for the momentary gratification of bodily needs. Yet Diderot does not place Rameau's nephew in some larger sacred history. Rameau's nephew readily admits his vices, but even "Myself," the Philosopher, is uncertain whether those vices have any consequences beyond this life. At the end of the dialogue, we are left wondering if Rameau's nephew had anything at center that defined his being and gave direction and meaning to his life. Diderot was willing to pose the possibility that human beings did not have immortal souls, indeed, that they might have no souls at all.

CONCLUSIONS

Diderot marks a threshold; beyond him lies the modern world, Nietzsche's nihilism and Freud's somatic mind. My purpose has been to suggest ways of conceiving of a human life less familiar to us. I do not wish to propose that any of these authors should be normative. Rather, I would like to call attention to the variety of ways people of the past have conceived of what constitutes a human life and the richness of each one's definition of what it is to be human. For each, every human being was unique: whether one takes up Plato's notion of individual souls seeking knowledge of the Good through many different bodies; Augustine's understanding of *conversio,* in which the reorientation of each soul takes place at a different moment in a life and each soul pursues its longing for God along a different path; Dante's vision of all the different kinds of human frailty and love; Montaigne's speculation that each life is experienced through a different body, and that that experience defines human life; or even Diderot's characterizations of human beings united in seeking to allay hunger, but differentiated by the pantomines, or the "positions," they would adopt in pursuit of satiety. For all of these authors, the definition of human life was carried out over time by each individual human being, and guided by inner lights of differing orientations and desires. For all, human life comprised not only a body, but a psyche, a soul, or a mind. For four of them, human life was defined within eternity; the life of the organism did not define human life.

The following essays take up the biological event of the moment of death and the many different cultural and religious responses to death. In the first section, doctors offer often anguished thoughts from their perspective as those who most often witness death, those who are increasingly left to serve alone as society's witness to the passing of lives. In the second section, historians, an anthropologist, theologians, a literary scholar, and pastors speak of the different ways that cultures and religions articulate a frame of meaning for death, first as those religions and cultures locate death within a larger understanding of human life, and then as each has given form to grief, in funerals, in rites of mourning, in graveyards, and most recently, in the AIDS Memorial Quilt.

But let us remember each *life* as we address death and the art of dying.

Each life has its own definition, its own reference points, its own orientations and yearnings. Each patient understands death differently, according
to his or her religious and cultural traditions; for each of them, death's
meaning depends not on the organism, the human body, but on how each
conceives of life. For many, if not most, it is life that frames death and gives
it its meaning, its place. We do not know if the soul is immortal, if there is
an eternity after death. We do not know if death is a portal or merely a
terminus, an end. But to speak of "terminal illness" is to define the life in
terms of the organism—it is to miss the quality and the character of the
living that continues to define that life. Socrates still speaks to the limits of
our knowledge:

> For let me tell you, gentlemen, that to be afraid of death is only another form of
> thinking that one is wise when one is not; it is to think that one knows what one
> does not know. No one knows with regard to death whether it is not really the
> greatest blessing that can happen to a man; but people dread it as though they
> were certain it is the greatest evil; and this ignorance, which thinks that it knows
> what it does not, must surely be ignorance most culpable (Plato 1954, 60).

Notes

1. The epithet "Divina" was added to the title in the 1555 Venetian edition.
2. I recognize the anachronism of this form of identity for much of pre-modern history.
Nonetheless, it serves to designate the geographical boundaries of the works I discuss.
3. In 1988, the great liberal I. F. Stone published *The Trial of Socrates,* in which he sought
to reconstruct the final days of the fifth-century Athenian (Boston: Little, Brown). In the
end, Stone condemned the Athenian democracy for its failure to support Socrates's right to
free speech. Although Stone did impressive research, reading widely in various Greek accounts, and called attention rightly to Socrates's "rough speaking," he remained profoundly
anachronistic in his understanding of Socrates's efforts to offend the jury at his trial. Stone's
view of Socrates partook both of the modern conception of the individual as autonomous
within democracy and of the biological model of human beings.
4. This canto is at the center of the entire *Comedy,* defining the principle by which the
whole is organized.

References

Alighieri, Dante. 1959. *The Divine comedy of Dante Alighieri.* Trans. J. D. Sinclair.
New York: Oxford University Press.
Augustine, Saint. 1984. *Concerning the city of God against the pagans.* Trans. H.
Bettenson. Harmondsworth, Eng.: Penguin.
Diderot, D. 1956. *Rameau's nephew and other works.* Trans. J. Barzun and R. H.
Bowen. New York: Bobbs-Merrill Library of Liberal Arts.

————. 1972. *"Le neveu de Rameau" et autres dialogues philosophiques.* Paris: Galli-
mard.
Montaigne, M. de. 1957. *The complete essays of Montaigne.* Trans. D. M. Frame.
Stanford, Calif.: Stanford University Press.
Montaigne, M. de. 1965. *Les essais de Michel de Montaigne.* ed. Pierre Villey. Paris:
Presses Universitaires de France.
Plato. 1954. *The last days of Socrates (Euthyphro, The Apology, Crito, Phaedo).* Trans.
H. Tredennick. Harmondsworth, Eng.: Penguin.

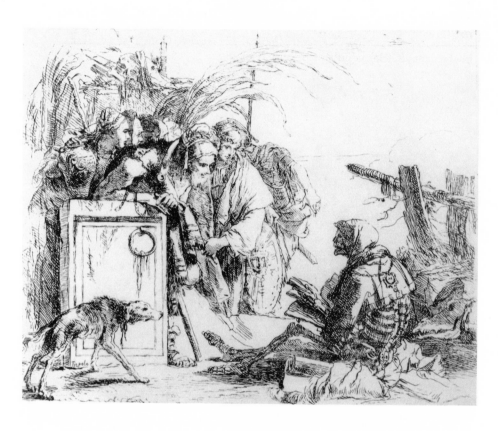

Giovanni Battista Tiepolo, *Death Gives an Audience (Der Tod gibt Audienz)*. Courtesy Graphiksammlung "Mensch und Tod" der Heinrich-Heine-Universität Düsseldorf.

Part 1 Witnessing Death: The Medical Battle

Introduction

Mary G. McCrea Curnen and Howard M. Spiro

Although doctors and nurses describe death and dying from a largely technical, biological viewpoint, their anguish is evident in the first part of this book. Lee Wandel provides an anodyne in her insight that defining life requires acknowledging death. American society is becoming—we are grateful—multicultural; but for now Western customs still rule our emotions and responses, and that is why her chapter brings the reader back to those Western traditions that have been responsible for what most of us think. So beguiled by scientific and technical prowess over the past hundred years are they that medical care workers forget how little human nature and character have changed over the centuries. Physicians can read what Harvey thought about the circulation of the blood with amusement, but Shakespeare still gives the keys to envy, lust, love, ambition, and even solace for some of the pains of the people we treat. The trouble comes when medical students and residents learn about the progress of medicine and not enough about what the past teaches the present.

From Wandel's graceful reminder, the reader moves to the medical battle, where hospital residents are the foot soldiers in the conflict with death, with many horror stories to tell. In the cause of cure, doctors and nurses have now to do so many things to elderly patients who might have been their parents or teachers—and to the young who might have been their friends—that they quickly harden themselves. Ill prepared for the intensive care units in which they must train and work, young physicians are not yet ready to comprehend how different is death at seventy than at thirty or forty. Eric Krakauer is an exception. A philosopher before he became a physician, he relates in sorrowful detail how three of his patients died and how that process affected them, their families, and the doctors and nurses taking care of them. His essay shows how philosophy can bring passion back to the medical task and how poetry and compassion make medical experiences far more human.

Peter Selwyn, deeply involved in the AIDS plague, recounts his emotional experience as a resident and young physician, struggling against the untimely death of so many patients.

In his reflections on death and dying, Sherwin Nuland tells how once he mistook action for thought, brilliance for compassion, and how fascination with biology and pathophysiology led him—and many of us—to forget the first duty of the physician: to relieve suffering. As the reader will soon discover, Nuland's message is one of hope, calling for more human medicine and more humane dying.

Is relieving pain helping patients to die? Alan Astrow wrestles with that dilemma to conclude that killing patients, with the goal of helping them by euthanasia, is morally unacceptable, whereas relief of suffering is praiseworthy. For many physicians and nurses, however, Astrow points out, the problem comes in the common belief that withdrawing "life support" is "killing" the patient, when to the contrary it is the disease that kills. So-called life support systems simply prolong their dying. Not all will agree, but all will learn from his meditation.

A pediatrician and ordained minister, Alan Mermann recounts from that double point of view how medical students learn to care for those who are suffering when they are paired with a very sick patient. He fears the ambiguous feelings of doctors who must confront suffering; the protective loss of their emotion and empathy may turn compassionate medical students into hardened physicians.

James Kenney offers a classical interlude of other meditations on death and dying and reminds us how much we as nurses and doctors have to learn from the past and from our writers and poets.

From her long experience in caring for children with cancer, Diane Komp tells us how she found faith in attending to her young patients. Children have their own ideas of death, but Komp urges caregivers "to find the words that frame a merciful version of truth." She stresses the role of spiritual beliefs and insists on the parents' right to talk about death with doctors and nurses. Those who treat dying children must learn that in facing death children fear mostly separation and isolation.

New Haven's popular pediatrician Morris Wessel gives an account of his long experience caring for children who have lost a loved one. Keeping children away from funeral services, however well intentioned, proves traumatic for many youngsters because it takes them away from family at a time when they need to be closer than ever. The sad questions of a child at death require the understanding, comfort, and support Wessel helps us to give when they mourn.

Once Dean of the Yale University School of Nursing, Florence Wald put her heart and career into establishing the first American hospice for the dying at the outskirts of New Haven. With Ed Dobihal, then the hospital chaplain, and many others, Wald gave death a new setting and thereby a way to die more humanely. In her account we read how all of us can help during those last days.

Joanne Lynn has also learned much from her experience in caring for the aged. She gathered numerical data on their probability of survival, their activities, their cost of care, and more. This information is invaluable for improving our present health care system. She comments that in our time we'll probably die of a chronic illness, but we probably will have no one who acknowledges that death is approaching, manages it, or helps us with it: "it is easier to get open-heart surgery than Meals on Wheels. . . . antibiotics than eyeglasses, and . . . emergency care than to get sustaining and supportive care."

Alan Novick closes this first section, Witnessing Death, with a memoir of life in the gay community, the first community in the United States to be ravaged by AIDS. His poignant words tell of the losses and of the pain and anguish this epidemic has cost him and those he loved.

This section truly makes us witnesses to death and lets us contemplate the problems that medical care workers encounter. The reader may be bewildered at how little most doctors attend to the spiritual needs of their dying patients. That is why the editors planned the second section of this book: Framing Death. There, cultural and religious considerations in caring for the dying will be discussed in a way that enriches and informs our understanding of death.

Chapter 1

Attending to Dying:
Limitations of Medical Technology
(A Resident's Perspective)

Eric L. Krakauer

In the past half-century, the primary site of death in our culture has shifted from the home to the hospital (Ariès 1974, 87–88). Nurses and residents have displaced family and friends as the primary tenders of the dying and witnesses of death. The practice of sending the gravely ill to the hospital to die now has become standard. Yet it is not at all clear that the dying are usually best served when they are sent to an acute care hospital, and within the hospital to an intensive care unit.

This "displacement of the site of death" from the home to the hospital has occurred without anyone planning or intending it. This societal trend has occurred not by design but rather because of the irresistible movement of technological development: as technologies of all sorts, including life support and organ replacement, become available, we as a society seem to find it unthinkable and immoral not to use them. This movement has brought humankind many dilemmas: our desire for safety and health has brought us overpopulation, weapons of mass destruction, and pollution, thereby threatening our safety and health. Our desire for longevity and freedom from suffering has drawn out the process of dying from hours or days to months or years and may considerably worsen suffering. The unplanned final stages of this unexpectedly long process of dying often now occur in acute care hospitals poorly designed and staffed to provide comfort care to patients and support to their families. Residents in particular are badly trained for this task. In short, although we as physicians attend to the dying every day, we have not attended to dying itself, to the process of dying in the technological age.

Because residents are poorly prepared to attend to dying patients, they sometimes feel resentful for being forced to do so. We are often uncertain as to how aggressive our treatment should be, uncertain as to how best to approach the patient or family with this question, and sometimes even uncertain as to the appropriateness of raising this question with a distraught family or obtunded patient. When DNR (do not resuscitate) and DNI (do not intubate) orders have been agreed upon and written, uncertainty often still remains as to how to administer comfort care. Medical students and residents are trained primarily to diagnose and treat acute illness, and they naturally take this as their principal role. Harried residents can therefore become resentful when each day patients arrive for admission who are chronically ill, whose conditions will never improve dramatically, who may die soon no matter what is done, and yet for whom aggressive acute care is expected.

In what follows, I will give three examples from my own experience as a medical student and resident of how we attend to dying patients, examples that manifest our fundamental inattention to dying. I will then offer some thoughts on a previous, "tamer" mode of dying and on what might be done about the current "wild" state of technological death (Ariès 1974, 14).

CASE I

Medical postponement of death often subjects patients to considerable violence and results in significant suffering. This is what Callahan calls "the violence of technological attenuation" (1993, 34). This violence can be brief and extreme, as in cardiopulmonary resuscitation, or protracted over months and years. The death of Mr. G, a forty-four-year-old man, illustrates both types of violent technological attenuation of death.

When I was called urgently to see Mr. G in the cardiac intensive care unit, he had already been an inpatient for ten months. Probably about one-third of the medical house staff had participated in his care at one time or another. For the previous six months, he had required intensive care to support his badly failing heart as he waited for a transplant. For eleven weeks, he had required an intra-aortic balloon pump to augment the feeble pumping activity of his heart. This device kept him completely immobilized on his back with a large catheter protruding from the major artery in his groin. Living, or rather, dying (for him, the two were the same) in the alien technological wasteland of the intensive care unit, he was even more removed from his home community, family, and friends than are other hospitalized patients. In addition, in spite of all his medications and the balloon pump, Mr. G continued to suffer from chest pain and severe anxiety. This was his status quo as he awaited a new heart and the possibility of a new life.

Around 6 P.M. one evening when I was the resident on call in the cardiac intensive care unit, a cardiac arrest alarm was called. It was Mr. G, and as a transplant candidate, he was a "full code." The standard resuscitation was initiated. Because Mr. G had no pulse, chest compressions were begun. Because he was not breathing, he was intubated by inserting a large tube into his windpipe and connecting this to a ventilator or breathing machine. And because he had only limited intravenous access, large needles were inserted into his veins. Over the next four hours, Mr. G's pulse intermittently disappeared and returned two or three times. By the time we were able to maintain a pulse and a modest blood pressure with very powerful medications, his breast bone and ribs were fractured in multiple places from the compressions. The heart surgeons were called in the hope that Mr. G's dire situation would place him at the top of the New England transplant list and that a transplant could be done emergently. But no suitable heart was available. Recognizing that Mr. G's heart would very likely continue to arrest until he could no longer be resuscitated, the surgeons elected to take him to the operating room to implant a left ventricular assist device: a small pump designed to take over part of the heart's function transiently until a transplant can be done. In the morning, after the heart-lung bypass machine was turned off, Mr. G could not sustain a blood pressure even with support from the assist device, the balloon pump, and multiple medications, and he died. When I broke the news to the resident in charge of his care, we both cried, not so much I think because Mr. G had died, but because of the torture he had endured for naught.

CASE 2

I have just alluded to the difficulty sometimes of discussing "do not resuscitate" orders with the patient and family. All too often, a situation arises where house staff and attending physicians agree that resuscitation in the event of cardiac arrest would be futile and unreasonable, but the patient or family steadfastly insists on a "full code" status.[1] Physicians may not want to put a patient with widely metastatic cancer, facing a painful death, through the added pain and violence of resuscitation. They may feel that a patient in a persistent vegetative state is essentially no longer alive and should be spared the indignity of resuscitation. They also may not wish to resuscitate a conscious patient who has no hope of leaving the intensive care unit, even if a resuscitation were successful. In each case, physicians may feel that such patients would be done a terrible disservice if they were resuscitated. Patients and families, on the other hand, may have many reasons for insisting on resuscitation. Sometimes even families with a thorough understanding of the violence and futility of resuscitating their loved one may still opt for resuscitation for religious or other reasons.[2] Physicians must be very careful to respect the customs and beliefs of patients from religions and cultures different than their own and to not impose their own values on their patients. Nevertheless, physicians sometimes find it appropriate to request DNR status from the family. When families are resistant to the univocal request of the medical team for DNR status, there is often a breakdown of trust or understanding between family and physicians. The case of Ms. S illustrates this point.

Ms. S was a fifty-three-year-old African-American woman with a severe cardiomyopathy causing end-stage congestive heart failure. She had been admitted to the medical intensive care unit for respiratory distress requiring intubation and intravenous vasopressors to stimulate the heart and improve circulation. While in the intensive care unit, she had multiple episodes of cardiac arrhythmias and received cardiopulmonary resuscitation. She was painstakingly weaned from the ventilator and from vasopressors twice, only to have recurrent respiratory distress and hypotension, which necessitated reintubation and reinstitution of vasopressors. Her mental status had progressively deteriorated. Even when she was off the ventilator, not sedated and most awake, she did not know where she was or what year it was. She clearly could not appreciate her situation. It also became obvious that Ms. S would never be able to leave the intensive care unit. The house staff were upset about having to put her repeatedly through the ordeal of intubation and resuscitation. The attending physician, an exceptionally caring and sensitive person, agreed that further resuscitation would be futile and unreasonable, and asked the family for DNR and DNI status. The family refused initially and remained steadfast in their refusal, even after many hours of meetings with the attending physician and house staff.

This case illustrates, I think, a lack of trust and understanding between physicians and family, exacerbated by a certain cultural difference. First, several family members were clearly distraught over the critical illness of Ms. S and may have been psychologically resistant to the suggestion that further resuscitation would be futile. This sort of resistance often weakens with time. Moribund patients and their families often also fear that if they agree to DNR status, they will be "deemed unworthy of further attention" and "abandoned" (Schneiderman 1994, 112). This fear probably can be assuaged by careful reassurance that intensive *comfort* care will be provided. Better public education about futile medical treatment and about alternative comfort care would make such discussions easier. The cultural difference that complicated matters in this case was that between working-class African-Americans and upper-middle-class European-American physicians. Here, the terrible American legacy of enslavement and systematic disenfranchisement of African-Americans by white America may still manifest itself in the understandable though regrettable suspicion that European-

American physicians may not have the best interests of their African-American patients at heart. The most honest, well-meaning, and patient discussion may not be enough to overcome this barrier erected over centuries, although every effort ought to be made until the day when such distrust disappears.

At the family's request, Ms. S remained a "full code" until inflammation around her heart caused by kidney failure made it useless to perform chest compressions. She died finally in the intensive care unit as all her major organs failed.

CASE 3

While hospice programs may provide excellent and appropriate care for the dying, most social and medical institutions are still ill equipped to do so and many health professionals do not know how. Talk about dying (and dying itself) is taboo not only in society at large; serious discussion about care of the dying has been far too rare even within medicine. This is why Ariès speaks of the "hushing-up," "displacement," and "forbiddance" of death in contemporary United States culture. The poor terminal care given Mr. K, one of my first patients as a medical student, illustrates Ariès's point.

Mr. K was a twenty-seven-year-old HIV-positive man who walked into the emergency department one day complaining of shortness of breath. He was found to have a very low level of oxygen in his blood, probably because of a pneumonia. He was admitted and treated with oxygen and antibiotics, but his respiratory status continued to deteriorate. He was transferred to the intensive care unit, intubated, and mechanically ventilated. Even in the intensive care unit he did not improve. His chest X rays appeared worse, indicating the accumulation of fluid throughout his lungs, and he required ventilation with 100 percent oxygen for adequate oxygenation. Pure oxygen, however, is toxic to the lungs and will destroy them within days. Efforts to decrease the fraction of inspired oxygen below 100 percent failed because his blood oxygen level dropped precipitously each time this was tried. He was agitated and required high doses of a sedative to calm him. After five days on the ventilator, his lungs indeed developed oxygen toxicity. It was clear that he could not survive and that the ventilator was deferring for a short while the inevitable. With the family's consent, he was made DNR.

At that point, the intensive care unit team called the floor team intern who had admitted Mr. K and with whom I worked to announce that they were transferring Mr. K out of the intensive care unit and back to the ward, in effect to die. It became then the intern's job to discuss this with the family and to ask their permission to turn off the ventilator. The harried intern hastily called the family together and bluntly laid out the situation. He allowed little time for discussion. The family consented to turning off the ventilator. The intern wrote the order and hurried off to look after his other fifteen patients. The family was invited to visit Mr. K, still heavily sedated, in his room for a few minutes only. After they left, a respiratory therapist removed the ventilator as ordered. Predictably, this left Mr. K gasping for breath.

Observing from the nurses' station, I saw that Mr. K had simply been left alone to die. One of the nurses who had taken care of Mr. K during prior admissions noticed this as well. We both put on masks (tuberculosis was still a possible diagnosis at the time) and went into Mr. K's room. Nurse N sat down at the bedside, took Mr. K's hand, stroked it gently, and spoke soothingly to him. Tears ran down her face. I stood behind her with my hand on her shoulder, fighting back my own tears. Mr. K's gasps became less frequent and violent. After thirty or forty minutes, they ceased altogether.

In a sense, Mr. K was indeed abandoned by his physicians when death became imminent. This is precisely what many dying patients fear. Once it was ascertained that he could not survive, he was discharged by the intensive care unit team and his care was turned over to general medical physicians and nurses who were too busy with their many patients to provide intensive comfort care to a dying, ventilator-dependent patient. The family was then suddenly confronted with unfamiliar physicians at the moment of their most difficult decision and greatest grief. They were not invited to stay with Mr. K as he died. To my knowledge, adequate doses of morphine to prevent the sensation of suffocation were not given, perhaps because this was not felt to be necessary in a patient who was sedated and only minimally responsive to voice. This will remain for me an example of how never to treat a dying patient or a grieving family.

CHANGING WAYS OF DYING

These three cases illustrate what Ariès calls "wild" technological death. But death was not always so fraught with anguish and despair, so feared and detested that it was deferred as long as possible with life support technologies and hidden from view in intensive care units. According to Ariès, the millennium preceding the end of the Middle Ages was a time of "tame" death. Death was not fought against, says Ariès, but accepted calmly and easily as each person's Destiny (1974, 13, 25, 28, 103–4). No rigid distinction was made between life and afterlife, and the transition from one to the other evoked "no great show of emotion" (12–13, 104). Death was made into a ceremony in which everyone participated. "The dying man's bedchamber became a public place to be entered freely. . . . It was essential that parents, friends and neighbors be present" (12). In marked contrast to present custom, children were invariably brought to the bedside. Death was neither pitiable nor frightening, and it did not need to be hidden. It was merely the crossing of an important generational "threshold," which like other crossings such as marriage was made into a public ritual.

In the sixteenth and seventeenth centuries, the development of a new scientific world view brought about change in Western attitudes toward the body, health, and death. One of the most important engineers of this new world view, Descartes, wrote extensively on medicine. His work conceived of the human body as an object, a "machine" composed of parts that can be studied, examined, measured, and experimented with. It can also be "repaired," "managed," and "maintained" to keep it functioning well (Descartes 1981, 195). As Ivan Illich points out, this scientific conception of the body transformed birth, pain, disease, and death into technical problems best handled by physicians who are primarily technicians or engineers (1976, 146, 156, 184). Attempts to address our current uneasiness about how we care for the dying must proceed by way of a careful analysis of the origins of modern medical thinking, especially in the work of Descartes, Bacon, and Kant.[3] In *Medical Nemesis,* Illich makes an important contribution to this analysis.

As part of the Cartesian project of making "man" master and possessor of nature, the individual thinking human subject displaced God at the center of the universe. Henceforth, the world existed for the individual who perceived it. Both Illich and Ariès point out that the early development of this individuality and personhood may be seen in the changing attitudes toward death in the fifteenth century (Illich 1976, 177–204; Ariès 1974, 27–52). With the "predominance of serial time," symbolized by the proliferation of clocks, came a new sense both of personal identity and of the "finality of personal death" (Illich 1976, 179, 180). Death had become a "natural force," and it could therefore be mastered like any other natural force. In the first century of printing, one of the most common types of books printed was the guidebook or practical manual for mastering every aspect of life, including death. The first of these was called *Ars moriendi,* or *The Art of Dying.* The human body was itself no longer sacred and inviolable, but open to invasive exploration by dissection (Illich 1976, 184–86). Rembrandt's *The Anatomy Lesson of Dr. Tulp* (1632) appeared virtually simultaneously with Descartes's *Discourse on Method* (1637), in which he posits that scientific, experimental medicine can not only cure "an infinitude of maladies both of body and mind" but also possibly even free us from "the infirmities of age" (Descartes 1981, 120). For Descartes, humankind can do

God one better. Scientific medicine can overcome the worst shortcoming of God's greatest invention, the machine that is the human body. This shortcoming is its mortality. Death itself can be mastered.

TECHNOLOGICAL DEATH

Illich sketches a history of this endeavor: the medical prolongation of life. By the eighteenth century, the ability to defer death was attributed to physicians, and this attribution gave them new economic and social status (Illich 1976, 191–93). Henceforth, a "natural" death came to mean death under medical care from a medically certified disease. In the eighteenth and early nineteenth centuries, this kind of death was the privilege of the middle class, who could pay for medical services. By 1900, however, death under medical care was claimed as a right by the labor movement (Illich 1976, 194–95). Illich suggests that this universal demand for "equal consumption of medical services" was, and remains to this day, counterproductive because it displaces more appropriate concern about pathogenic social conditions. People have become so concerned about receiving their fair share of medical services that they ignore the possibility of eliminating the causes of many diseases that make medical care necessary. We also have come to ignore to a great extent the possibility of dying in circumstances other than under intensive medical care. We have largely given up the right to determine how and when we will die by ceding this right to the medical system. As physicians within that system, the care we provide dying patients is determined too much by the diagnostic and therapeutic technologies available. This is demonstrated, I think, by all three cases I have described. Mr. G and Ms. S were kept alive for long periods in intensive care units under extraordinarily stressful and painful circumstances. In Mr. K's case, once all available technologies of acute care and life support had been tried and proven unsuccessful, he was virtually abandoned. In contemporary medicine, technology often seems to control us more than we control it. The result is what Illich calls "administered" technological death, and the indignity and violence of this death are precisely what Ariès calls "wild."

It is now widely recognized that technological medicine, for all its sophistication and power, has made no great advances toward mastering death. On the contrary, in Callahan's words, death is now "harder to predict, more difficult to manage, the source of more and more moral dilemmas and nasty choices, and spiritually more productive of anguish, ambivalence and uncertainty" (1993, 33). What is not widely recognized, I think, is the depth and complexity of the problem of attending to dying. Callahan calls for medicine to make death more "peaceful" by expecting, preparing for, and accepting death; by desisting from the "violence" of "technologically attenuating" death; and by choosing instead the proper "combination of treatment and palliation" to make a peaceful death possible (34). Certainly, medicine can and must do better at palliative care. But the changed and accepting attitude toward death for which Callahan calls does not take seriously enough the scientific, objective view of the world and of ourselves, which is fundamental to modern Western thought. To truly give up the will to ultimate power over nature, and thus over death, the will to infinitely defer death, would be to call into question the absolute legitimacy of the modern objective mode of thinking. Heidegger, in his late work, explores this crucial but enormous task.

Descartes's legacy, according to Heidegger, is that all that is, all beings, including human beings, are conceived as objects. Every thought redetermines the meaning of Being or what it means to be, namely, an object of thinking. All objects, objects *as such,* and thus all beings, are masterable by thinking. For Heidegger, technology is much more than the products of thought with which we go about mastering nature. Thinking is itself technological because every act of thought reconceives of the world as objective and thus masterable. If we are to begin to resolve our perplexity about death, our apparent inability to attend to dying in spite of our great technological power, we must take seriously Heidegger's point that thinking is itself a "mastering objectification" (Heidegger 1977, 149, 150). Heidegger's late work on technology makes no call for a return to some impossible pretechnological, pre-objective thinking. Rather, it demonstrates that modes of thinking and ontologies are themselves historical, and it thereby opens the possibility of thinking otherwise. Heidegger attempts to prepare for an alternative mode of thinking by retracing the origins of thinking as mastery in the history of Western philosophy.

The road to a less inimical and domineering attitude toward nature and death may therefore be very long and arduous; it may demand a reevaluation of fundamental Western values and a reexamination of the entire Western intellectual tradition. Short of this, however, what can we do today about our apparent inability to attend well to dying?

TOWARD MORE HUMANE ATTENDING

A few voices can now be heard offering concrete suggestions for more compassionate and intelligent care of the dying. These authors emphasize that palliative care that "maximizes comfort and dignity for the patient and for the grieving family" (Schneiderman 1994, 110–14) may require an intensity, aggressiveness, and ingenuity rivaling that of an intensive care unit (Saunders 1982, 1169–71; Wanzer 1989, 844–49). The patient must continually be reassessed to make sure both that pain is adequately controlled and that the patient and family do not fear abandonment. Pain and suffering must be treated until they are relieved and by any means necessary, even at the risk of side effects including sedation, respiratory depression, hypotension, and death. As long as the intent is pain relief and the patient does not clearly choose pain over sedation, all of these side effects are acceptable. Intensive comfort care also includes keeping the patient clean, good skin care, controlling nausea and vomiting, welcoming the presence and involvement of family and friends if desired by the patient, and attention to the psychosocial and economic stresses that may burden both patient and family (Wanzer 1989, 847). Toward these ends, clergy, nurses, social workers, psychiatrists, surgeons, and physicians must coordinate their efforts. Finally, comfort care must be recognized as one of the most important services that medicine can offer, and it must therefore take its place among the other major disciplines taught in medical school and residency. When all of this occurs, perhaps residents will feel less uncertain about how to care for dying patients and less resentful of them. Perhaps patients will no longer fear abandonment, and families like Ms. S's will find less cause to distrust physicians. These measures will not resolve medicine's dilemma of how to deal with death. They will, however, help us to avoid doing inadvertent harm to our most vulnerable and needy patients.

Notes

1. For good discussions of the concept of medical futility, see Jonsen 1994, 107–9; Schneiderman et al. 1994, Schneiderman et al. 1990, Tomlinson and Brody 1990, and Truog et al. 1992.
2. A notable example of this sort of preference is the case of Helga Wanglie in Minnesota. Cf. Angell 1991, 511–12; and Miles 1991, 512–15.
3. Cf. Jecker 1991, 5–8.

References

Angell, M. 1991. The case of Helga Wanglie. *New England Journal of Medicine* 325 (7): 511–12.

Ariès, P. 1974. *Western attitudes toward death from the Middle Ages to the present.* Baltimore, Md.: Johns Hopkins University Press.

Callahan, D. 1993. Pursuing a peaceful death. *Hastings Center Report* 23 (4): 33–38.

Descartes, R. 1981. *The philosophical works of Descartes.* Trans. E. S. Haldane and G.R.T. Ross. New York: Cambridge University Press.

Heidegger, M. 1977. The age of the world picture. In *The question concerning technology*, trans. William Lovitt. New York: Harper.

Illich, I. 1976. *Medical nemesis.* New York: Bantam.

Jecker, N. 1991. Knowing when to stop: The limits of medicine. *Hastings Center Report* 21 (May–June): 5–8.

Jonsen, A. 1994. Intimations of futility. *American Journal of Medicine* 96 (2) 107–9.

Miles, S. 1991. Informed demand for "non-beneficial" medical treatment. *New England Journal of Medicine* 325 (7): 512–15.

Saunders, C. 1982. Principles of symptom control in terminal care. *Medical Clinics of North America* 66 (5): 1169–83.

Schneiderman, L., K. Faber-Langendoen, and N. Jecker. 1994. Beyond futility to an ethic of care. *American Journal of Medicine* 96 (2): 110–14.

Schneiderman, L., N. Jecker, and A. Jonsen. 1990. Medical futility: Its meaning and ethical implications. *Annals of Internal Medicine* 112 (12): 949–54.

Tomlinson, T., and H. Brody. 1990. Futility and the ethics of resuscitation. *Journal of the American Medical Association* 264 (10): 1276–80.

Truog, R., A. Brett, and J. Frader. 1992. The problem of futility. *New England Journal of Medicine* 326 (23): 1560–64.

Wanzer, S., D. Federman, S. J. Adelstein, et al. 1989. The physician's responsibility toward hopelessly ill patients. *New England Journal of Medicine* 320 (13): 844–49.

Chapter 2

Before Their Time:
A Clinician's Reflections on Death and AIDS

Peter A. Selwyn

This brief essay has a much more personal tone than the scientific papers that I have written about AIDS, because I have come to understand that it is precisely through one's own relationship with death and loss that a physician can be most helpful to patients who are facing AIDS and other life-threatening illnesses.

I graduated from medical school in June 1981, the same month and year that the first cases of AIDS were reported by the Centers for Disease Control (CDC). In a brief description that appeared in the *Morbidity and Mortality Weekly Report,* the CDC reported several clusters of cases of Pneumocystis carnii pneumonia and Kaposi's sarcoma in young homosexual men in New York and California. It was not evident to the CDC at the time, and certainly not to me as I went forward from my medical school graduation, that this new disease, later to be called AIDS, would become the leading cause of death for young adult men in the United States by the end of the decade. It was even less evident to me, with my belief that I had acquired in medical school the knowledge to serve as the foundation for my medical practice, that this disease, which was not known when I began my training, would soon become the major focus of my work as a physician.

I began my medical training at the end of the historical period that John Arras, my former colleague at Montefiore Medical Center in the Bronx, used to refer to as the postwar "Pax Antibiotica." Infectious diseases had become apparent vestiges of the prescientific past, and the ability of medicine and technology to conquer disease—in the true military sense of the word—seemed limitless. When death occurred, it happened either to the very old or, less commonly, to the very young. AIDS profoundly changed all this.

In 1984, when the first wave of the AIDS epidemic was just beginning to overwhelm the vulnerable population of drug injectors in the South Bronx,

I took a position as the medical director of Montefiore's drug abuse treatment program there. It felt as if we were witnessing the arrival of the plague, as tens and ultimately hundreds of patients became critically ill and quickly died from this disease whose course we could do very little to affect. Unlike the few of my earlier patients who had died of other causes, these hundreds of patients were virtually all in their early thirties, almost all of them within five years of my own age. They also included many women, some of whom I attended during pregnancy and the birth of their children. These young families seemed to represent some sort of terrible anomaly in the usual patterns of the life cycle, an anomaly in which death seemed to have crowded out life and cruelly and painfully destroyed the family, often over generations. These events were particularly compelling to me since the pregnancies of my wife and the birth of our two children occurred during those same years. I would sometimes share stories with the women about my wife's pregnancies, the birth and early development of our children, and then watch helplessly as these same women became ill and died, sometimes preceded by their infants. For the uninfected children, orphans of the epidemic, we began to see a steady stream of grandparents, themselves often weathered by life and their own struggles, coming forward to care for them after having watched their own children die of AIDS.

Surrounded unexpectedly by so much suffering and death, I was for a time oddly unaffected by it emotionally. I felt a strong need to be doing this type of work, although I could not have articulated what this need was about, and I found a great satisfaction in being with my patients. On a certain level, however, something was missing for me. After working in this environment for several years, one day I attended a concert at the Cathedral of Saint John the Divine in New York, near Columbia University. As I was leaving the church after the concert, I noticed an area along one of the side walls where many candles were burning on a small table, in front of a plain white scroll. On the scroll, in calligraphy, were the simple words, "In Memory of Those Who Have Died of AIDS." I stopped and stared at these words, and suddenly began to cry for all of the patients I had lost, whose faces I could see through the flickering light of the candles. I realized then that this work was about me and my life in ways that before then I could not have understood.

Elisabeth Kübler-Ross, who has been one of my most important teachers, has said, "You never cry for anyone else, you only cry for yourself." After my experience in the cathedral, I came to understand the meaning of this simple phrase. My own father died suddenly at the age of thirty-five when I was eighteen months old, either in an accident, or, more likely, by suicide. Because of the unusual circumstances of his death, this event and even the memory of his life quickly became family secrets that I was not permitted to discuss, so in effect I experienced a double loss. It was not until over thirty years later, when I was confronted with all the deaths of these young men and women, whom I could do little more to save than I could have saved my father, that I began to realize how I had never come to terms with this first and primal loss. This realization became a gift for me as I then began the work of grieving both for my father, which I had never done, and for all of my patients who had died. After going through this process, I found that I became better able to be with my patients in their pain, to support them without feeling the blind compulsion to rescue them from something from which there was no rescue, and to stay with them as they approached death without feeling that I had somehow betrayed their trust.

I have learned that the greatest gift that I can give to patients is to allow the awareness of my own pain and loss to deepen my solidarity with them as they face their illness and death. I am now convinced that it is the physician's fear of death, and his or her own unexpressed grief, that are the biggest impediments to true empathy, and result instead in pity, despair, revulsion, and the kind of numbing detachment that finds refuge in technological interventions and narrow medicalization.

I do not wish to indulge in the romanticization of death, nor in imagery of the nobility of dying young. I cannot sit and listen to a young father, as he bargains with God to be allowed to live long enough to dance with his eight-year-old daughter at her wedding, without feeling the crushing sense of injustice that permeates this disease. Indeed, it has been very gratifying to me, and a great relief as a clinician, to experience the dramatic advances in the medical care of people with AIDS over the past decade. These advances have affected the clinical course of HIV infection in profound ways, and helped to convert a fulminant and rapidly fatal illness into a more chronic and treatable, albeit incurable, disease.

Nevertheless, I can recall with a kind of wistfulness the simple and unencumbered nature of my relationships with patients at an earlier time in the AIDS epidemic. Before our current therapies even existed, we coexisted with patients in the grim but complete knowledge that all that physicians could do was to be there, to bear witness, support, comfort, and accompany patients through their illness. What enabled, or even entitled, us to do this was simply our commitment not to abandon the patient and our experience in traveling this road with others before. I believe that this fundamental connectedness with the patient best characterizes the history of the physician-patient relationship over the centuries, until powerful forces over the past decades fragmented and distorted it, often in the name of specialization, expertise, or increasing technical sophistication. At times it has been disturbing to observe how the rapid introduction of medical interventions for AIDS—which, thankfully, have increased in number and complexity in recent years—has resulted in some ways in the tendency to over-medicalize the disease and lose sight of the important fundamental dynamics of life and death that still ultimately define it. I can only hope that the advent of the therapeutic era for AIDS, while eagerly awaited, does not have as a consequence the loss of empathy and the doctor's willingness simply to *be* with the patient, when instead one can find solace or distraction in pharmacological protocols and technological tinkering.

It has always seemed ironic to me how those who are confronted with dying are much more aware of living, and, in some cases, able to live in a much more immediate and intense way than those whose daily lives are dulled by the unconscious assumption that time is unlimited. Many patients have told me that having AIDS has allowed them, required them, to dispense with all of the superficial distractions and wasted energy that take up so much of our attention, and has led them to focus on what was truly important in their lives. One patient said to me, "AIDS is kind of like life, just speeded up." This anecdote describes well the accelerated process in which, over a period of weeks to months, people with AIDS may have to confront issues in the life cycle that normally would have taken years to decades: the deaths of peers and family, the loss of physical and sexual functioning, deterioration in cognition and memory, and the effects of aging on one's bodily appearance. Another patient once remarked, with a little bitterness but also some satisfaction, that AIDS had taught him who his friends really were. I remember yet another patient, a thirty-six-year-old late-stage AIDS patient, who had been using intravenous drugs for over twenty years and for the first time in his life had been able to stop. Confronting death had enabled him to undergo a spiritual conversion, stop using drugs, and reconcile with his family. Shortly before he died, he told me that he was thankful that he had finally learned what it was like to live in the world and experience life without being addicted to drugs, and was only sorry that he had to die in order to do so.

Ultimately, for both patients and physicians, AIDS is about letting go. Only through a process of letting go of fear and blame, and through an acceptance of our own vulnerability and powerlessness, can we become truly powerful. Only in this way can we, as the great labor organizer Mother Jones put it, "mourn the dead and fight like hell for the living," and go beyond the artificial distinctions between physician and patient to get on with the process of living and dying that all of us have to confront. Elisabeth Kübler-Ross has said, "Nobody gets out of this life alive." I think the avoidance of this reality often impedes physicians' ability to be effective in truly caring for their patients.

I often recall my last conversation with a patient in her early thirties whom I will call Maria. She had been ill for several years and seemed to be lingering on well past the point that anyone thought she would survive. She had a six-year-old daughter, whom I will call Lisa, who was being cared for by her aunt because Maria was already too weak to care for her. The aunt had agreed to raise the child after Maria's death, which helped relieve Maria's concerns but made her feel guilty that she was leaving her only child. In fact, it became clear that this was the only reason she had survived as long as she had. She felt that she needed to die, but couldn't. She was also saddened because Lisa was angry with her at times for not being able to play with her and not being there to put her to bed at night. Finally, when I asked Maria what she was most afraid of, she said that she was afraid that by dying she would be betraying her little girl, that this would somehow be a sign to the child that she didn't truly love her. After we talked about it, she came to realize that these two things were totally separate; she had to die, but nothing could ever take away the bond between her and her daughter. I encouraged Maria to talk to Lisa about this and to let her know that she would always love her and always be with her in her heart, no matter what happened. The next day Maria spent the whole day with her child, and said everything that she needed to say. Two days later, she died, peacefully, at home.

For me, the thirty-nine-year-old physician, with the eighteen-month-old boy inside who had never had that last conversation with his father, nothing could have been more gratifying.

Chapter 3

The Doctor's Role in Death

Sherwin B. Nuland

If Eric Krakauer can properly call his chapter "Attending to Dying," perhaps mine should be entitled "The Attending *in* Dying." There was a time when the perspective of the attending physician was really quite different from the resident's—it had to do with the number of years in practice, the wisdom acquired during those years, and perhaps a more mature outlook on life. I think those days are gone forever. I remember Elisha Atkins saying to me one day that there are no longer any professors of medicine, there are only super chief residents. That is very much the way I feel about all of us who are involved in teaching young people the highly technological aspects of medicine that they have mastered so very well, thanks to the example (in many ways a poor example) that we have set for them.

Every man likes to think of himself as Everyman. On the other hand, every doctor likes to think of him- or herself as unique: "No one has ever been a doctor like I have been." I'm going to try to tread a little bit of a middle ground here and present myself as Every Doctor. I want to relate how I went astray and how it is that attending physicians and professors have become super chief residents. They have become so excited by the pathophysiology of the disease process and by attempting to solve what I like to call The Riddle of disease that the paramount problem facing them is no longer the problem of relieving the human tragedy with which they are faced in intensive care units, on the wards, in their offices, and perhaps in homes.

I went into medicine for the same reasons as did so many doctors of my generation. Actually, these reasons were no different than those for which the present generation, and I like to think future generations, did or will go into medicine—namely, that I had in my mind an image of a man (in those days when almost all doctors were men) who, when he arrived at our house at a time of crisis, gave us the sense that everything was under control even if that specific problem could not be solved. His presence meant that someone was there who would understand just what the family of this very sick person needed at that time. That was the kind of man I wanted to be. So, like so many of my generation (and present and future generations), I applied to medical school to become that man.

And what happened to me? The same thing happened to me that has happened to virtually every young man (and now woman) who has gone to medical school for those and similar reasons: I became, by the time I was a third-year medical student, fascinated with the process of disease and increasingly with technology. There was not a lot of technology in the 1950s, but advances through subsequent decades were ever more complex and awe-inspiring. In recent years, I have watched countless medical students go through this same evolution. They become so intrigued by the kinds of things they can do with their hands and their minds—and increasingly with machines—that they want to be more and more like their "super chief resident" professors just as I had wanted to be ever more like my own professor of cardiac surgery.

By the time I was a senior in medical school, I was no longer someone who thought that the greatest good I could achieve was the relief of human suffering. Instead I had begun to believe that the greatest good I could achieve was the solution of The Riddle of disease. To me the paramount objective was to understand the disease process so well that I could imagine what was going on in the abdomen. In this way, when the operation took place I already had absolutely predicted what I would find; then of course I could predict my ability to see to it so that it would be cured permanently. The person who came to me with that abdominal disease remained someone for whom I felt empathy, compassion, and kindness, and I provided the sort of professional politeness that I felt was required. But during my six years of training, my role models became the fast-moving senior residents who seemed so brilliant in the operating room and at diagnosis. My secondary role models became my attending physicians. Of course, my attendings were kind and they were professionally polite, but these qualities were simply vehicles that they used to treat the disease that so fascinated them.

I write this not to condemn either myself or the physicians of my or a later generation: after all, we must remember that to those attitudes we owe the extraordinary accomplishments of twentieth-century medicine, specifically American medicine, which is the envy of the world. Had this transformation not occurred among so many young people, we would have a more humane medicine, but we certainly would not have a medicine capable of the miraculous things that we see in intensive care units, operating rooms, and oncology units every day. And so it has been a double-edged sword for American and Western medicine that those of us who went into the field somewhat fascinated by biology or pathophysiology became ultimately so completely taken in by it that we became less and less concerned with what I believe and have always believed is the ultimate job of medicine: the relief of suffering.

One of the first things young doctors learn as they watch their attending physicians, senior residents, and others whom they are trying to emulate is that we must never allow our patients to lose hope. So when we find ourselves in situations where we are in the midst of highly technical pathophysiological matters of diagnosis and therapy, we still remember that we must leave our patients with the message that there is hope. But the arrogance of the message that we really leave is that hope must come, and can only come, from *us*. In our modern medical culture, we physicians actually believe that the hope that can come to a patient with a serious, lethal, or terminal disease is the hope that only the doctor can give.

I have consistently been as guilty as other physicians of this arrogance of believing that the hope I can give is that there will be, when things look darkest, a light that will provide weeks or months of life, if not actually a cure.

I would like to think that we can reorient American and Western medicine to a broader concept of hope—one that includes sources of hope other than the physician. As Eric Krakauer has pointed out (quoting the work of the social historian Philippe Ariès), medicine has taken death and turned it into something that belongs only to physicians. We have medicalized death, which is part of the general sanitization of death that seems to feed so well into the needs of American society. We have now cleansed death and hidden it. The term "hidden death" comes up repeatedly in the work of Ariès. Society and medicine have conspired to turn death into something that belongs to the medical profession.

Here let me become autobiographical again. I have four children, born in two platoons. Two were born in the 1960s, and two were born in the 1980s. When the first two were born, I sat outside the delivery room like every other father and chewed my fingernails until the delivery was announced. But when my second two children were born in the 1980s, they were delivered by a midwife, with an obstetrician nearby. The deliveries were in the hospital, but they were done in what was called a birthing bed, which is basically just a regular bed. The midwife's proud assistant was me. There was an enormous difference between those two experiences, a difference similar to that which Eric Krakauer described. He called attention to the difference between the experience of death during the sixteenth, seventeenth, eighteenth centuries and the deaths we see today. The medical profession did not cause the change in childbirth practices; rather the American and Western European public did, with the women's movement. The women's movement took back childbirth from the doctors and pointed out that it is really part of the life cycle. Childbirth is not a disease—childbirth is something that belongs to the family. It can be helped by physicians, but is not ultimately a medical phenomenon. I would propose to you that death is not a medical phenomenon either.

The classical term *euthanasia* means "good death." In the latter part of the nineteenth century, when syringes had been developed and after morphine had been synthesized from opium, doctors were expected to provide euthanasia in the sense of easing a patient comfortably to the eventual, natural good death. This is the way I conceive of the role of physicians in the immediate and longer term. Physicians should be supporters of traditional euthanasia—good death. Death primarily belongs to the dying. The only really significant event that occurs at the time of death is the death itself, not medical attempts to subvert it. In our attempts to prolong life, we often prolong dying. Further, the chief actor in the drama of death is the person who is dying, and not the would-be rescuer, who is in reality a groundling in this drama.

So how does this discussion leave us with hope? What kind of hope can we as family, and as physicians, provide people who are facing the virtual certainty of their own death? Eric Cassell, in his wonderful book *The Nature of Suffering* (1991), points out that hope is intimately connected to the future. A loss of hope means in essence that one feels that his or her future is lost. We act on the vain concept that death takes away the future, that the future of the dying individual is lost. I would argue that this is not necessarily so. One does not need to believe in an afterlife to believe that there is a future for those who are dying and that there is hope in visualizing that future. As I look over the definitions of hope, I find many meanings, but only one universal: hope lies in the expectation of a good that is yet to be. For the dying person, this means that some good can yet be snatched out of the tragedy that appears as the immensity of death or the loss of the future.

What can that hope be? Of all the kinds of hope a doctor can give his or her patient at the end of life, several encompass all of the rest: there is the hope manifest in the promise that the patient will not suffer unnecessarily; the hope inherent in the certainty that he or she will not die alone; and the hope that comes from knowing that each dying person will live on in the minds of those whom he or she has loved.

A major factor in my perspective, which I didn't fully appreciate until about ten years ago, is that increasingly, as specialized physicians, we do not know our patients very well. Patients come to us at the onset of a disease, and the more highly specialized we are, the more critical is the point at which patients reach us. We almost come to believe that their life histories start when they step into our offices or when we meet them in the emergency room or an intensive care unit. Obviously that is not so. One of the reasons that I make a plea in my book *How We Die* for the renewal of the concept of the family physician is that at the end of life, when faced with distressing decisions, a patient should have with him or her a longtime counselor who understands his or her values in addition to medicine. Insofar as possible, physicians should be able to guarantee that a patient's values will be respected, and a patient should know that there will be no unreasonable attempts to prolong life. I don't believe that the super-specialists of today are capable of making those kinds of commitments to patients they hardly know.

What other kinds of hope can there be? There is, of course, the clearly spoken hope, wish, and promise that no one will die alone. The figure frequently given is that 80 percent of us will die in hospitals or long-term care units. Of course, dying in such a place doesn't necessarily mean that one dies alone, but we know that all too often attempts to prolong life seem to prolong certain kinds of anguish, because in doing so we, as super-specialists, can continue to believe that we may yet effect a cure.

What we need is a new orientation by doctors who take care of the most serious diseases in our hospitals. They must develop a self-image that encompasses not only the physician who fights disease, but also the doctor who, at a given point, helps patients to die peacefully and serenely.

As physicians, we abandon our patients too frequently, and almost universally. I attribute this failure again to our fascination with The Riddle of disease. It is the riddle of diagnosis and therapy that captivates us. When we realize that there is no longer anything we can do, the very stimulus that has made us excellent doctors in an intensive care unit is lost: we lose interest in our patients as individuals because we have lost our interest in their now insoluble Riddle. We must reorient ourselves to an image of us not only as enemies of disease but also as people who stand by the values that brought most of us into medicine—the values that inform us that our primary mission is to relieve human suffering.

There is another kind of hope that anyone can give, not only physicians. This other kind may be the most important hope, in fact. As I become older, I become ever more convinced that the things that are really important in our lives don't have anything to do with winning prizes, getting into medical school, or the worldly rewards that we see about us. The most important things in life really are those that we all share—things like births in our families, weddings, baptisms, confirmations, bar mitzvahs, and yes, even the time when we die. At the end of life, it is our obligation as physicians to those who are dying to bring some understanding of what their lives have meant to us. This, it seems to me, is the most important form of hope: when a person dies, the ideals that he or she has represented to the few who have been most important in life will not die but live on. The values will live on. The kinds of things that that person represented will live on in us. This is what I mean when I use the word *immortality*. And the hope that they will indeed live on in the values and lives of those with whom they have been close can be an enormous source of hope for dying people.

I had originally intended to close with an excerpt from *How We Die*. Somehow it seems much more appropriate to cite a single sentence—and not from a book I wrote, but from another, *Precepts*, composed almost two and one-half millennia ago by Hippocrates. It is the message that I would like to leave to members of the health professions, and to others: "Where there is love of humankind, there is love of the Art of medicine."

References

Ariès, P. 1981. *The hour of our death*. New York: Knopf.
Callahan, D. 1993. *The troubled dream of life*. New York: Simon and Schuster.
Cassell, E. 1991. *The nature of suffering*. New York: Oxford University Press.
Katz, J. 1984. *The silent world of doctor and patient*. New York: Free Press.
Nuland, S. B. 1994. *How we die: Reflections on life's final chapter*. New York: Knopf.
Quill, T. E. 1993. *Death and dignity*. New York: Norton.

Chapter 4

Thoughts on Euthanasia and Physician-Assisted Suicide

Alan B. Astrow

As I write this, a second cousin, aged eighty-two, lies comatose on a ventilator in the intensive care unit of a large public hospital in New York City. He had had a mild stroke and then was suddenly stricken three weeks ago with what appears to have been a brain stem stroke. While now unresponsive to all stimuli, he still has minimal activity on a brain scan and so has not met the criteria for brain death. His physicians believe that the likelihood for recovery is near zero, but because he has never explicitly stated his wishes regarding how he would want to be treated in such circumstances they will not remove him from the ventilator. (His closest relative would consent to removal.) He is now also on tube feedings and on intravenously administered antibiotics for pneumonia.

My cousin's fate, suspended between life and death, captures for me the missing dimension to discussions about assisted suicide and euthanasia. Although these topics arouse strong emotions, I see them as peripheral to the care of most dying patients. As a practicing oncologist and hematologist, I have cared for many patients dying from cancer. Legalization of assisted suicide and euthanasia would do little, in my view, to enhance the comfort of these patients and would threaten substantial public harm and damage to the morale of the profession. I see instead two central problems in our treatment of the chronically ill and dying: (1) the failure to acknowledge that the patient is dying and that comfort is the most appropriate goal, and (2) the misuse of high technology in a manner that prolongs the dying process.

My cousin does not require a statute legalizing euthanasia to be allowed to die in peace. He only requires that our profession and our health care institutions resolve to withdraw intrusive medical technology with the family's consent when that technology serves no human purpose. I serve on the staff of a Catholic hospital where, accompanying a tradition of hostility to active life-taking, a strong aversion to the delivery of futile or nonbenefi-cial care usually leads to the withdrawal of ventilatory support in cases like that of my cousin. I suspect that there is considerable public confusion in this area, that an outlook that holds life sacred is mistakenly seen as requir-ing endless life support.

In my own field of medical oncology, one frequently encounters the related problem of aggressive treatment continued past any realistic hope of benefit. Dying patients are sometimes identified with their tumors, and continued "attacks" by chemotherapy and radiation therapy may prolong rather than relieve their suffering. I agree with Daniel Callahan that it is precisely the "obeisance to medical technology" that has led to the fear of a "technologically induced bad death" and spurred public support for physi-cian-assisted suicide (Callahan 1994, 13–15). Doctors and patients together need to face our finitude openly and acknowledge the limits to curative medical interventions. Suffering and death are parts of life that we rightly struggle against but ultimately have to accept. Angry disillusionment may follow an overly optimistic assessment of modern medicine's power. As a result, our approach to incurable illness may focus unnecessarily on the extremes of treatment without limit and at all cost or, alternatively, a swift clinical end. Expanded access to hospice services and improved training of doctors and nurses in comfort care for the dying might reassure patients and their families that they need not confront chronic progressive illness alone.

ASSISTED SUICIDE: NOT THE ANSWER

The argument for physician-assisted suicide and euthanasia rests on those cases of chronically ill patients who can find comfort nowhere but in death. As an oncologist I too have treated many patients whose uncon-trolled tumors have produced intractable pain, profound nausea and an-orexia, foul-smelling discharges, and worse, for whom death could be seen only as a blessing. In most instances, though, a withdrawal of active medi-cal treatment combined with unstinting use of analgesics and sedatives to control symptoms allows the patient to die comfortably and peacefully. Western religious traditions acknowledge the principle of "double effect": treatment intended to relieve the suffering of a person with advanced incurable disease is morally acceptable even if that treatment secondarily shortens the person's life.[1] There is an inherent ambiguity in the care of the dying, and the line between relief of suffering and end of life is often blurred. I wonder at times whether most physicians understand that pro-viding adequate doses of morphine to control pain and suffering for a dying patient is not considered "killing" but instead represents symptom relief within the best traditions of medicine (Cleeland 1994).

I have certainly treated patients who, it seemed, died "too slowly" despite my efforts to provide for their comfort. One such patient with head and neck cancer and advanced liver metastases wasted away over a three-week period while on a morphine drip, to the great distress of his family. A nurse who knew the patient but had not been directly involved in caring for him later told me that had we been more attentive to his grimaces we might have increased the rate of his morphine drip more quickly. This sort of teamwork offers the best hope for relief of suffering in dying patients. Team members can work closely with the patient and family to forestall conflicts, avoid moral crises, and share the emotional burden that these inherently troubling situations carry.

Some patients who are depressed and discouraged by the prospect of lingering physical decline but are not yet "actively dying" want an end to their suffering and assistance in ending their lives. I think here of some patients with Lou Gehrig's disease (ALS), Alzheimer's, stroke syndromes, or AIDS. We can all understand these wishes; none of us can be sure how we might respond to such grim prospects. At the risk of sounding callous, nevertheless, I believe that physicians should not honor such requests. While we are obliged to respect the desires of patient and family, the choice of death over life cannot be viewed as just another choice if medicine is to maintain its moral stature. The patient's prerogative must be exercised within the framework of generally accepted standards of physician conduct (Annas 1994). Killing, even for the best reasons, has generally been seen by physicians as unprofessional and immoral.[2] Most physicians, aware of the uncertainties of medical decision-making, the strain of caring for the chronically ill, and the hostile feelings that such patients may engender, understand the need to accept limits to what a physician is empowered to do. I agree with Leon Kass (1992): were physicians to attack life directly, we would "contradict the inner meaning of our own profession." To put physicians in the role of judging the appropriateness of a person's request to end his life can only further "medicalize" a fundamental life experience whose meaning has already been diminished by the dominance of medical technology.

We need to consider the impact of legally sanctioned and professionally monitored suicide on the public morale as well. Persons who wish to end their lives can usually find the means to do so. In facilitating that choice by granting professionals a license to kill, however, we all become complicit in an antisocial act. The reduction of end-of-life decision-making to a matter of private choice threatens to reinforce the isolation of the chronically ill and their families. How we die carries with it a profound meaning not only for the dying person, but also for all those who have loved and cared for that person. Often, suicide provides only the illusion of a solution to the fundamental human problems of disappointment, suffering, and death and simply transfers the burdens and conflicts at the end of life to the loved ones left behind.

The stricture against active life-taking carries with it a communal obligation to support those suffering from serious illness. Sickness and death should serve as constant reminders of our common bonds and need for one another. A seriously ill and disheartened person may overcome despair and rediscover meaning and purpose in life. We need to encourage those efforts on a personal level by not turning away from people with incurable illness and on a social level by helping them continue to work and maintain their positions within their communities. We also need to assure the incurably ill that, when all else fails, we will provide for their comfort.

In persons with end-stage ALS, for instance (at substantial risk, say, of choking on their own saliva), I would think it medically and morally proper for a physician familiar with the patient to provide morphine for comfort. In contrast, I believe that to have euthanized that same person, even with the person's consent, six months earlier in the course of the illness—or for a stranger with an M.D. to poison that person with carbon monoxide—would be murder.

If we were to evaluate the recent case in Michigan that led to Dr. Kevorkian's acquittal, the case of Thomas Hyde, a thirty-year-old with ALS, it would be important to know what options the patient's own physicians had offered him. What made him turn to Kevorkian? We need to look past the headlines to understand how patients with ALS are cared for as they approach the end. We all hope for a cure for ALS and other chronic degenerative diseases, but in our search for cure, are we neglecting individualized and thoughtful care?

My stance provides no easy answer for the extreme cases where it seems that despite our best efforts to provide symptom relief, a patient may, in the words of Lonny Kliever (1993) of Southern Methodist University, "suffer himself to death." One could, for example, imagine the plight of a person left quadriplegic after a cervical spinal cord injury who, after prolonged consideration, decided that he did not wish to go on living but did not have the ability to induce his own death. Kliever has argued that the traditional objection to suicide did not anticipate the modern-day "prolongation of the living-dying interval" achieved by medical technology. Where serious illness would once have brought a relatively quick end to a person's suffering, medical "advances" allow people to live for long periods of time with chronic debilitating illnesses, sometimes against their will. Arguing from a Methodist perspective, Kliever has suggested that our religious traditions ought to rethink their aversion to assisted suicide to reflect contemporary conditions. I would respond that if medical technology is doing more harm than good for a patient, we physicians should not hesitate to withdraw that technology with the patient's consent and while seeing to the person's comfort.

Both the public and caregiving professionals need to confront our self-contradictions in this area. Our actions toward the chronically ill often belie our rhetoric. The medical care system, fragmentary and technology biased, encourages physicians to focus on the performance of lucrative technical procedures. There is little glory in caring for a suffering human being. Reimbursement formulas favor high-intensity curative care so that, for example, bone marrow transplantation is a winner for financially strapped hospitals, and hospice is a loser. Pain control for dying patients may be ostensibly a major public concern, but in practice it carries a lower priority than the "war on drugs." In the same states where editorialists demand the legalization of physician-assisted suicide, the Drug Enforcement Administration harasses physicians who provide appropriate narcotic pain medications for cancer patients. With the provision of comfort care for the incurably ill so often lacking, it follows that assisted suicide and euthanasia are seen as cheap and easy solutions.

REALISTIC HOPE

An honest appraisal of what medicine can and cannot do will be central to any efforts to improve care of the dying. In the field of cancer treatment, for example, despite all the genuine advances and the promise for the future, large numbers of our patients die and will continue to die of their disease. Sherwin Nuland (1994) has protested movingly against giving false hope to cancer patients and their families. "I never had a single experience in which an oncology consultation did not result in a recommendation to treat," he wrote in *How We Die*.

While Nuland overstates the case—in my experience many, if not most, oncologists are honest and caring physicians—his broader point has merit. The field as a whole has been advertised in a way that creates unrealistic expectations in the public's mind. We have made giant strides in earlier and more accurate diagnosis of cancer and in our understanding of the molecular mechanisms of oncogenesis and metastasis, and we have also achieved striking success in treating several of the less common malignancies such as Hodgkin's disease and the non-Hodgkin's lymphomas, childhood leukemia, and testicular cancer. Nevertheless the outlook for the vast majority of cancer patients has changed little over the past sixty years. In 1990, half a million Americans died of cancer, 23 percent of all deaths.

The sad contrast between the promise of our contemporary scientific approach to cancer treatment and the reality of unhappy outcomes in so many of our cancer patients promotes misunderstanding, catastrophic disappointment, and anger. Patients are often sent to medical oncologists when surgeons and radiation therapists have exhausted all other options. The patients come with the hope that we will enable them to live, not help them to die. Often the referring doctors create false expectations to relieve their own burden of guilt. Or they might rid themselves of an "unsuccessful case" by delivering a harsh prognosis, leaving the patient emotionally devastated. The setting of achievable goals is undermined, and open engagement with patient and family becomes a lonely and draining pursuit. In the absence of effective support, the patient with progressive incurable cancer may be subtly encouraged simply to end it all.

Let me illustrate. A woman in her sixties was referred to me by an internist colleague. She had complained only of a cough, but after diagnostic evaluation an unresectable biliary tract cancer was found. Two days before her first scheduled appointment with me, she saw a well-known surgeon from the cancer center across town who told her that there was nothing that could be done. The woman canceled her appointment with me, and the next day I was told by her internist that she had been found dead in her apartment.

Such experiences have reinforced my conviction that physicians are ill equipped to decide whether a person's life is worth living. The ability to offer realistic hope to a person with a critical illness is a subtle art that not all physicians possess and that even the most skilled have difficulty sustaining. The diagnosis of incurable illness presents the patient with both a physical and a spiritual crisis. People suddenly confront long evaded questions of meaning and purpose. What does it mean to be alive? Why go on in the face of incurable illness? Rather than function as judge and executioner, the physician could serve as a crucial moral presence in this setting, a source of strength and courage.

Open discussion of these sorts of existential issues within the profession and amidst the public at large, along with frank acknowledgment of the limits of medical technology, may help us to clarify values, achieve public consensus, and improve the care of the dying. I agree with Christopher Lasch that medicine has ill served the public and itself by focusing excessively on technique. "Like other professions," Lasch has written (1991), "medicine has been uncomfortable with its role in shaping public opinion, preferring to address itself to the technical problems it feels qualified to solve. But its silence on the broad ethical questions that govern popular expectations leads the public to expect far too much of medicine and create painful and now familiar situations in which doctors themselves are expected to decide questions of life and death."

Even as we physicians own up to our shortcomings in this area, we have reason to be hopeful. There is far less shame and secrecy in the care of cancer patients, for instance, than was the case thirty years ago. The success of Nuland's book testifies to the public's hunger for truthfulness in the care of the dying. Conferences like the one that inspired this book break through the silence within our profession. The growth of the hospice movement, as well as recent decisions of public figures like Jacqueline Kennedy Onassis, who chose to die at home, and Richard Nixon, who elected to forgo invasive life support, are also encouraging signs of a new public awareness of limits. Even the movement to legalize physician-assisted suicide, while I disagree with its goal, has served to focus public attention on the treatment of the incurably ill. The New York State Task Force on Life and Law has issued a two-hundred-page report on physician-assisted suicide. I suggest that the next step we take should be to move from ethical reflection to an investigation of social reality. Perhaps a national study on the care given to those at the end of life is called for. If we doctors are to eschew suicide as a solution, we will have to understand the true needs of the progressively ill and act, as a profession and as a society, to address them.

Notes

1. Dr. Timothy Quill, a leading proponent of the legalization of physician-assisted suicide, has questioned the usefulness of the principle of double effect, viewing it as an "idealized ethical perspective" that fails to acknowledge the full range of our motivations in our treatment of the incurably ill. He asks that we become "more forthright and explicit about our motivations and responsibilities" and openly admit that we sometimes intend our patients to die (Quill 1993). I am unconvinced by this argument. While it is certainly true that all human actions are the product of a mixture of motives, conscious and unconscious, and while the acknowledgment that there are patients for whom death would seem like a relief may paradoxically help sustain our relationship with a suffering patient, it does not follow that it is appropriate to act on every motive, of which we become aware. A degree of self-knowledge is central to skilled physicianship. The principle of double effect reminds us that we must respect limits. If we sense that the predominant motive for a treatment is the desire to end a person's life, rather than to provide comfort and relieve symptoms, we need to pull back. Of course, we are ultimately judged by our actions, not by our thoughts, and Quill is right that the intent behind our actions is often ambiguous. Still, as a practical matter, reasonable people can and must make distinctions, even while granting the physician the benefit of the doubt in trying circumstances. Dr. Kevorkian might claim in court that he did not intend to kill his patients, but it's hard to construe his particular set of practices in any other way.

2. The Hippocratic Oath states: "Never will I give a deadly drug, not even if I am asked for one, nor will I give any advice tending in that direction."

References

Annas, G. J. 1994. Asking the courts to set the standard of emergency care: The case of Baby K. *New England Journal of Medicine* 330 (21): 1542–45.

Callahan, D. 1994. The Sanctity of Life Seduced: A Symposium on Medical Ethics *First Things* 42: 13–15.

Cleeland, C. S., R. Gonin, A. K. Hatfield, et al. 1994. Pain and its treatment in outpatients with metastatic cancer. *New England Journal of Medicine* 330 (9): 592–96.

Kass, L. R. 1992. Why doctors must not kill. *Commonweal,* no. 2 (Sept. 8), special supplement.

Kliever, L. D. 1993. Must we suffer our way to death? Religious warrants for active euthanasia. Unpub. manuscript, Park Ridge Center for the Study of Health, Faith, and Ethics, Park Ridge, Ill.

Lasch, C. 1991. Letter to author.

Nuland, S. B. 1994. *How we die: Reflections on life's final chapter.* New York: Knopf.

Quill, T. E. 1993. The ambiguity of clinical intentions. *New England Journal of Medicine* 329 (14): 1039–40.

Chapter 5

Learning to Care for the Dying

Alan C. Mermann

> It hath been often said, that it is not
> death, but dying which is terrible.
> —Henry Fielding, *Amelia* (1751)

Skills vary in their importance and power. We are in awe of the surgeon who reassembles a hand or replaces a heart valve, and learning to do that work requires time and an intensity of dedication that are admirable. Many aspects of medical care involve similar expertise: the psychiatric interview that deftly and gently reveals the intricacies of a hidden life; the skillful obstetrical delivery that saves both lives; the trained ear that hears and correctly classifies the heart murmur. These accomplishments demand our profound respect. But the skills required may not reflect the inner life of the physician—that deep pool of feelings, relationships, desires, and loves in which we are immersed from the beginning to the end of life. For many doctors, professional life is often defined by work done with minimal interest in the patient as a person. There are many criticisms of physicians and our health care facilities, and I do not wish to add to them. But there is a widespread sense that physicians and surgeons are peculiarly distanced from patients' concerns about their diseases and treatments. The most difficult of these issues to discuss is of course death as the finale of that illness.

Can we learn to be receptive to these very personal concerns of others, to hear the exquisitely sensitive and intimate questions posed, and to offer support and kindness in a situation that we have not experienced ourselves? Can we be open to the unique nature of each person's life and relations, offering ourselves as coactors in such an intensely private and idiosyncratic drama? How do we learn to care for the dying in personal ways that are as skillful and significant as the clinical and research techniques we prize in the trained physician and investigator? Is there any hope that the days of our lives with others could resemble a time "when men and women seem by one consent to open their shut-up hearts freely, and to think of people below them as if they really were fellow-passengers to the grave, and not another race of creatures bound on other journeys" (Dickens 1954)?

Learning to care for others who are suffering and dying is similar to learning to love. If we are fortunate, we are exposed to love as a child and begin our journey through this life knowledgeable in the ways and means of loving: the awareness that others have needs; the willingness to make sacrifices for others; the concept of nurture; and that strange and astounding revelation that the more we give of ourselves, the more we receive. It is this latter point—the giving of ourselves—that I shall develop in the following discussion.

A close corollary to learning what it means to love is the enviable characteristic of the best of our caregivers—the ability to identify with the needs, concerns, and feelings of others. Identification with those who are ill can free us to give them the care and nurturance they require. To make the case that we can—indeed, must—learn to care for the dying, I shall recount my own experiences during the past decade with medical students, staff, and their patients.

MEDICAL STUDENTS

Two truths have emerged from [themes that recur in] my conversations with medical students and doctors, my readings in the extensive contemporary literature on "death and dying," and my own experiences as a physician and a chaplain: (1) we have remarkably ambiguous feelings as we confront suffering and dying in others, and (2) profound changes occur during the transition from medical student to physician. Many of us know the serious concerns and expressed sensitivity that entering students have for caring for those who are sick and perhaps dying. The dean of admissions is not the only one who hears these concerns; they are voiced frequently during the first two years of medical school. But something happens when medical students begin their clinical rotations. The house staff and the attending physicians, by personal behavior and conversation, underplay the significance of personal feelings and empathy in the care of patients, the very attributes students thought would characterize the good physician. The intimate and anxious questions that inevitably arise when a patient is threatened by serious disease are discounted in favor of discussions of the sciences and techniques of medicine and surgery; personal issues are labeled the concerns of nurses and social workers. The result is disappointment for both students and their patients. Students are often dismayed to realize that their initial idealism has been replaced in part by a learned detachment.

In an informative and engaging study of undergraduate and graduate students at Yale published in 1967 in the *Yale Journal of Biology and Medicine*, Kenneth Keniston, a psychologist, described three adaptive techniques that medical students use to respond to stress: "a propensity to counter, master, and overcome sources of anxiety, a tendency to react to stress and anxiety by an active effort to change the environment, and a highly developed ability to respond intellectually to troublesome feelings." When these adaptive techniques are applied to learning to care for the sick and dying, they can cause students to distance themselves from patients as people and to concentrate instead on their patients' therapies and other essential needs. A logical and seemingly necessary detachment from the personal issues in health care then becomes reasonable, indeed, inevitable.

Students' need to feel knowledgeable, competent, and skilled in treating seriously ill patients can, almost imperceptibly, lead to their becoming physicians whose training is superb, but whose responsiveness to the emotional, philosophical, and spiritual aspects of living and dying is limited. Will this learned response to the intensely private and individual feelings of others cause them to distance themselves from their own feelings as well? Suppression of feelings and emotions is one way in which doctors cope with the stresses of patient care, often to their loss (Mermann 1990). To separate oneself from fear and anxiety can be a distressing accomplishment for a doctor. Students may wonder what education has done to their earlier and professed concern for, interest in, and commitment to the personal welfare of the sick and the dying.

THE PHYSICIAN

In-depth communication with persons who are very sick is difficult, to say the least. Many physicians respond to this challenge by avoiding it, by devoting a minimum of time during patient visits to conversation about obviously central medical concerns. One reason for this avoidance may be that physicians have greater fears about death than many people; these fears may even be a reason some choose the profession. Some doctors see death as a defeat for caregivers dedicated to healing and well-being, as an implication that they have nothing to offer the dying. Doctors can also send subliminal messages that dying is not within the province of medical care. Of course, for all of us, caring for the dying triggers anxieties about mortality and contemplation of our own inevitable deaths.

Other disturbing observations have been made about the doctor-patient relationship. I am surprised at the number of angry doctors. They are angry about growing administrative and organizational constraints on their practices, about the uncertainties of the future of medical care in the United States, and in response to a proper concern for the millions of citizens with inadequate protection against the threats of serious disease. They are also angry with their patients. Their patients call too often, have questions that are difficult to answer, present issues that are not really medical, and ask for a degree of emotional support that can seem excessive. Doctors, for reasons not altogether clear, often send a message to their patients that their questions are importunate. The problem is that doctors receive inadequate training to answer these personal questions.

A central issue is the training physicians receive in *caring* for their patients. Medical education and residency training focus on the preservation of life, which is inarguably a most important function. As a result, however, preservation, not care, absorbs much of the time and effort of physicians responsible for the seriously ill and dying. This emphasis is of course related to the way in which death is identified with professional failure. Too often, little effort is expended on the personal role of the physician as listener and interpreter in the daily care of the sick. The good physician should be able to spell out the devastating effects of disease on our bodies with accuracy and compassion. Only if one truly appreciates the losses to be endured and understands the impact of irreparably damaged physiological functions can there be any hope for sympathetic care. To a person stricken by the announcement of a life-threatening diagnosis, this lack of this understanding—the retreat of the physician from the scene—is a catastrophic event.

THE PATIENT

The resilience and strength of persons with serious diseases are a remarkable testament to our determination to survive despite tremendous challenges and to do so with humor, concern for others, and a certain grace. Patients have much to teach us about the proper care of the sick, the damaged, and the destitute. They are excellent instructors because they know all too well the characteristics of the good doctor. If anyone knows the need for compassionate care, and how to provide it, it is the patient who is seriously ill.

How then do we teach student-physicians to be caring doctors? By watching a superior clinician interact with a patient, a student can learn to take an informed history, perform necessary examinations, and interpret laboratory findings—all with tact and evident personal concern for the total welfare of the patient. But it is finally the patient who can best teach us how to care for the sick. It is the patient's story, the patient's body, the patient's family, supportive or dependent—in short, it is the patient's life that is the central plot of the tale being told, the whole focus of our work.

Patients at university medical centers know that students have to learn from them: their histories, their bodies, their tests and treatments. Perhaps the most moving demonstration of this conviction is the donation of one's body to be dissected by first-year students, truly a gift so that others may learn.

Patients are willing and usually pleased to talk about the central personal facts of their lives as affected by disease. Obviously, tact, confidentiality, and sensitivity to privacy are essential for establishing a bond between patient and doctor. The devastation wrought by a mastectomy on a woman in our culture, with its tasteless and blatantly sexual advertising; the subsequent loss of hair from chemotherapy; and the presence of a portal vein catheter in the upper chest wall can be overwhelming to the patient. Knowledge of the significance of disfigurement must be a determining part of the physician's understanding of what it means to be a person. Understanding and accepting the power of definitive segments of our total lives, such as our sexuality, our memory, and our physical persona, are also required. The many insults to our physical integrity inflicted by disease and therapy affect our defining roles as parent, worker, and community member. How the doctor identifies with these losses and with adjustments made to them will characterize that physician's humanity as well as his or her professional skills.

There is a nearly absolute need for patients to trust their caregivers and to have confidence that they will not be abandoned as the disease advances. The fear of abandonment is powerful. Dying is all the more frightening if there is any possibility of it being endured alone.

If we can learn to care for the dying in ways that meet their medical, psychological, and social needs, we can bring about a remarkable change in the attitudes that flow both ways between patients and physicians. The onus for achieving this goal will rest primarily upon the education and training offered by medical schools and hospitals. The quality of this education in turn will depend on the skills of those who supervise and teach. In particular, there is an explicit need to help students understand the moral base that undergirds medical practice. There are time-honored principles for caring for others; spending our energies wisely; and assuming responsibility that can support us in our hours of discouragement. Instruction in virtue and values can help us change our perspectives, our techniques, and our understandings so that we can advocate and care for our patients at crucial hours in their lives.

LEARNING TO CARE

To help first-year medical students begin the long process of learning how to care for the seriously ill, I have developed a seminar whose goals are to "(1) learn to talk with, and listen to, sick persons; (2) learn to establish a professional relationship without the intrusion of friendship; (3) ascertain the meaning of compassion without sentimentality and the need for humility before the physician's ignorance; (4) learn of our common frailty as human beings, the finality of death, and the need we all have for companionship when death is near; (5) enrich the students' understanding of those in their care" (Mermann 1991).

Patients at the medical center, usually persons with cancer or AIDS, are interviewed as potential teachers. They are asked to commit to meet with students one-on-one, usually during clinic visits or while hospitalized, for the duration of the semester. An information sheet outlines the purpose of the course, my strict rule of confidentiality, and the potential benefits for both students and teachers. The course offers patients the opportunity to both recount their experiences with doctors in the management of their disease and describe the impact of serious disease on the whole of life. It is important for students to learn the varied mechanisms by which we cope with crises in our lives; how we manage, day by day, to live with a threatened future. There is a wide range of understanding among patients about their diseases, their prognoses, the hazards of various treatments, and expectations for their recovery or remission. Some want to know all details, others place their medical management completely in the hands of the staff. There is also a broad spectrum of religious, philosophical, and social beliefs that we affirm as persons, and these need to be heard by caregivers without judgment as we broaden our own thinking.

There are two introductory discussion sessions for students in the seminar during which filmed interviews are shown and a syllabus and reading materials for the semester are provided. I introduce the student to the teacher, and the education begins. I meet weekly with the students in small groups to talk about their ongoing experiences and to discuss ways of talking with others about serious concerns.

The students are usually anxious about starting the interview process. The patient-teachers are forewarned of this, and usually are quite adept at getting the dialogue going. In general, several interesting findings have surfaced over these past years. First, patients almost immediately grasp the purpose of the course, are pleased to have been asked to teach, and have a lot to say about the practice of medicine. Second, students are surprised at the willingness, even eagerness, of people to talk about their personal lives. A subtle, yet powerful aspect of these discussions is the dying patients' focus on living, not dying. This outlook surprises students who thought they were taking a course on "death and dying."

Third, we learn from the courage and resourcefulness of persons who are under extreme stress yet continue to think of others, of the future, and of the needs students have to learn more about the proper care of very sick persons. Students are given an opportunity to develop a profound sense of the meaning of the profession of medicine: scholarship, technical training, stability in times of crisis, and the willingness to sacrifice time and effort for the welfare of others because of the depth of understanding of human need.

Patients also confirm for students that we are all together on this journey from birth to death, requiring varied therapies for our particular devastations. For many, a life review defines a life that was lived with and for others. For some, a deep and abiding religious faith clarifies the final days of this life. For yet others, the opportunity to settle quarrels of the past, to seek and to offer forgiveness, and to focus finally on the mysteries of the self suffice to bring life to a peaceful close.

For the physician, care of the dying can enlarge a religious perspective on life. Many of us do not have a mature faith capable of sustaining us in times of exceptional stress. Students can learn from patients the varied resources that are used to support us when illness, loss, and death are imminent. Concerns for our spiritual life are real and particularly apparent when dying is a possibility. With education provided by patients who are carefully thinking through the relativity of faith to death, "the physician sensitive to the varied nuances of the life of the spirit can help to make this hour of transition a time of peace and acceptance" (Mermann 1992, 141).

In the religious tradition that we call Judeo-Christian, there are strong commandments to love God and one's neighbor. The Law and the Gospels state clearly that service is a necessary component of an active faith. Both the story of the Good Samaritan and the parable of the loaves cast upon the waters lay out our duties to serve and suggest the returns we can anticipate. We are confident that we shall be paid back many times for whatever we give. Those who invest of themselves in caring for the dying often comment on the value of the return on that investment.

The varied aspects of love can be used symbolically to illustrate these points. We brought nothing into this world, and we shall certainly take nothing out of it. Perhaps we shall be defined by how much of ourselves we give away to others who need us. As with love, we must give our ourselves if we expect to receive anything in return. This process requires work, commitment, education, some sacrifice of time and passion, and a distinct sense of identification with the sufferer. Also as with love, the richer the experience, the stronger the bonds that hold us to others and the more strength we shall have for sharing the burdens of others who, at the moment, are less fortunate than we. We cannot truly be the recipients of love without giving that love in return. The more we give of ourselves to others, the more we receive. We are constantly strengthened to sustain the other, knowing well that we will be needful in our own time. There is a commonality in this human venture that physicians are privileged to experience far more than many others. Our patients can teach us the depths and the heights of human life in all its intricacies, joys, and rewards. The role of the physician as a companion to patients on our common journey of life is enhanced when we realize that we have been gifted by them.

References

Dickens, C. 1954. *A Christmas carol.* In *Christmas books,* introd. by E. Farjeon. London: Oxford University Press.

Keniston, K. 1967. The medical student. *Yale Journal of Biology and Medicine* 39 (June): 349.

Mermann, A. C. 1990. Coping strategies of selected physicians. *Perspectives in Biology and Medicine* 33 (2): 268–79.

———. 1992. Spiritual aspects of death and dying. *Yale Journal of Biology and Medicine* 65 (Mar.–Apr.): 141.

Mermann, A. C., D. B. Gunn, and G. E. Dickinson. 1991. Learning to care for the dying: A survey of medical schools and a model course. *Academic Medicine* 66 (1): 36.

Chapter 6

Thoughts on Witnessing Death

James D. Kenney

*A*rs *Moriendi.* What a marvelous word *ars* is and how many different attributes it has. In the *Oxford Latin Dictionary, ars* takes up one page, with three columns. The first five definitions include professional, technical, and artistic skill; artificiality as opposed to the "ingenium" of nature; a trick wile or stratagem; personal quality or behavior; and a systematic body of knowledge.

What we as doctors deal with concerns almost all of these meanings of *ars,* as have many of the essays in this book. These multiple vantage points must certainly result from the complexity of the event of dying and the many people drawn into it—not just the patients themselves, but their families and friends, nurses, doctors, and clergy (not to mention the emerging culture of systems analysts, data controllers, "case managers," and electronic critics at measured remove).

I have some ideas and vignettes that are drawn from my own experience and conception of this very complex topic. With respect to the fact of death—of the termination of the life process—Eric Krakauer has already illustrated the reductionist view, which forever penetrates medicine. The electrocardiogram degenerates, becomes a tachycardia, then a fibrillation, and thereafter a straight line. There is chaos in the Purkinje cells, fractals go mad, and death follows. This is one view of the heart's stopping. It is rather more complex than simple cessation, and it has its origins not in a humane event but in electrophysiologic monitoring. It calls to mind an old and rather macabre bit of humor which was familiar to doctors of my generation: "The patient died in electrolyte balance." Everything had been done from a metabolic point of view; even though there might simultaneously have been various inadequacies and even errors, the numbers were right. Doctors are long since used to a reductionist viewpoint, and that influence has become ever more complex and more important.

In contrast, there is the often less informed view of the patient—though sometimes patients are quite sophisticated. Not long ago, a new patient said to me at the beginning of an interview, "I have had a B-cell non-Hodgkins lymphoma, which has changed from 75 percent expression to 5 percent. I have had a bone marrow transplant, and I have had Cytoxan infusions. In addition, I have had stem cell cytopreservation, and besides that I have had gene rearrangement studies." The patient was able to recite all of this detailed information without a hitch. There remain, however, much less informed viewpoints. The opening lines of a little poem by John Betjeman (1958) called "The Inevitable" provide an illustration:

> First there was putting hot-water bottles to it,
>> Then there was seeing what an osteopath could do,
> Then trying drugs to coax the thing and woo it,
>> Then came the time when he knew that he was through.

These first four lines contain three references to an illness that in the course of the poem we learn will separate the poet and his friend. Note that illness is twice referred to as "it" and once as "the thing" in the four lines. In this sort of circumstance the physician must become at least a moderator and translator.

Another excerpt from a poem concerns a farrier—a blacksmith—named Felix Randall, whose last stages of life are presented to us in the poem "Felix Randall" by Gerard Manley Hopkins:

> Who have watched his mould of man, big-boned and hardy-handsome
> Pining, pining, till time when reason rambled in it and some
> Fatal four disorders, fleshed there all contended.

While Hopkins has some degree of reductionist intent in discussing the notion of "some fatal four disorders," he does not get far into biology. The doctor, on the other hand, must reconcile contemporary science, and in addition the newly evolved apostolate of method for method's sake, with the concerns and realities of life and decline, and also with the mystery and complexity of death.

With respect to the beginnings of decline and the awareness of it, a poem by Po Chü-i entitled "Last Poem," written in 846 and translated in this century by Arthur Waley (1970), makes the point:

> They have put my bed beside the unpainted screen;
> They have shifted my stove in front of the blue curtain.

> I listen to my grandchildren reading me a book;
> I watch the servants heating up my soup.
> With rapid pencil I answer the poems of friends,
> I feel in my pockets and pull out medicine money.
> When this superintendence of trifling affairs is done,
> I lie back on my pillow and sleep with my face to the South.

One quickly appreciates that the poet is a cultured man, probably fairly well-to-do, who has been placed away from a more elegant part of his house and that he exists in an extended family. He is a person who has achieved a kind of psychological calm though he is aware of "inevitability."

Chaucer tells us about Troilus, who had been wounded and who said, in a nutshell, "Things aren't working out too well. I better get a doctor." He was, in fact, "an esy pacyent."

> Now lat us stynte of Troilus a stounde,
> That fareth lik a man that hurt is soore,
> And is somdeel of akyngge of his wownde
> Ylissed wel, but heeled no deel moore,
> And, as an esy pacyent, the loore
> Abit of hym that gooth aboute his cure;
> And thus he dryeth forth his aventure.
> from *Troilus and Criseyde*

His expectation was that a doctor would arrive and do well by him, certainly a legitimate and time-honored expectation.

Consider now some bedside experiences. Imagine a man, many years known as a patient, patrician, well over six feet in height, and long since accustomed to looking down at his doctor. When he began to decline from obstructive pulmonary disease, and was in hospital, he was severely short of breath and had great distress from bronchoconstriction. His doctor entered the room, and the patient, recumbent, pulled himself up on an elbow. He was in that moment revealed as deprived of his usual ecological niche, which was to look down at the doctor—a most distressing index of decline. The doctor, recognizing what was going on, sat down promptly and thereby eased some of the man's problem by getting to a different eye level. The doctor thus became a participant.

Consider also the case of a dear friend, with whom, when I was an undergraduate at Yale, I studied Italian informally on Friday nights along with four other classmates. (The pledge was that nothing, no matter how pretty she was, would interfere with our meetings.) We blitzed our way through the *Grandgent's Grammar*, and by the end of that half-year had managed to read the first canto of the *Inferno*. A dinner at Mory's celebrated the end of our efforts.

Many years later, it was my privilege to care for this same friend and teacher while he finally succumbed to urinary obstruction due to untreatable and widespread prostatic cancer. One kidney had totally ceased to function, and the other, still functioning in borderline fashion, was draining through a stent in his flank because a pelvic tumor completely blocked other outflow. He was sorely depleted, and his kidney was failing fast. Things reached a point at which once again the doctor sat down at the bedside. This time it was to say to an old friend, "I think it is time to stop." He agreed, and we did not pursue the matter in detail thereafter.

A few years ago when we opened the "new facility"—now the South Pavilion—of Yale–New Haven Hospital, Dr. Paul Beeson told of the last days of a colleague in Oxford. He recounted the death of his friend from hepatic cirrhosis and esophageal varices. Multiple procedures and a bed in an intensive care unit had led to a sort of imprisonment by technology. The man was bound down by tubes and wires and was made mute by an esophageal tube so that he was able only to wink at his wife when she visited during the intervals permitted. Dr. Beeson told us how he had admired the man's extraordinary courage in the face of these technological inroads, but then confessed that he asked himself, "What have we done to give this man such an awful way to die?"

Physicians can indeed provide an unfortunate excess of treatment. But remember that Chaucer's Troilus wants the physician to have the "loore" and to be current in his skills.

Thomas Browne, in the first part of the seventeenth century, always called the patient his "friend." He did not call him a patient:

> Now with my friend I desire not to share or participate,
> but to engrosse his sorrows, that by making them mine
> owne, I may more easily discusse them.
> —from *Religio Medici*

A truer word was never spoken. If the doctor does not know the patient, then he or she is dealing with something appropriate only for a record in a computer. The physician in the final analysis has to be the moderator, to guide not only the patient's relationship with "inevitability," but also the relationship of events and progress with family, nurses, house officers, and others. The rule that I keep in mind is simple rhetoric; one does things *for* people and not *to* them.

The first introduction I had to the circumstances and, if you will, the "style" of death was as a student in Boston doing an elective interval in Internal Medicine under the great Dr. Maurice Strauss. I recall presenting a case of a man with myxedema to him when a telephone call came in from New Haven. The caller told Dr. Strauss of the death of John P. Peters of Yale. I recall that Dr. Strauss said two things. One was, "I'll tell Bud and Bill" (Drs. Arnold Relman, then at Boston University, and William Schwartz, then at Tufts, two members of the extraordinary dynasty which Dr. Peters had begun). Dr. Strauss also asked, "Was it a kindly death?" I cannot ever forget his genuine solicitude.

The reason that I recollect these anecdotes is to reassure us that these qualities of care have been and still are available in the course of medical education. It is most important that the technology of management not remove the physician from his principal role. It is at present, alas, impossible for a doctor to take a ballpoint pen and write an order at Yale–New Haven Hospital. All orders are now a selection from a menu in a computer. That menu links us with cost accountancy—not with solicitude and certainly not with nuance. Add to this the presence and function of a non-physician "case manager," and sickness and death can seem to have their greatest relevance to payers.

Finally there is a subject that lies beyond electrophysiology, technology, and order sheets. The question about awareness of self and of soul has been raised by other authors in this volume. A few lines of an unnamed poem by the Emperor Hadrian, written long before the blossoming of the Christian era, tell of the Emperor's concern for his *animula*, his "soul," if you will, which someone else might refer to as his self or his ego.

> Animula uagula blandula,
> hospes comesque corporis,
> quae nunc abibis in loca
> pallidula rigida nudula,
> nec ut soles dabis iocos!

Note that he refers to the soul as the "guest and companion of the body." He wonders where it will go after he has died, becoming "all pallid and still and naked," and laments that it will not be able to crack jokes the way it used to. Hadrian certainly had a sense of self, and he had a distinct concern about what was going to happen to his "self." The same friend and mentor with whom I studied Italian, and whose case was discussed earlier, translated Hadrian's verse in 1976 as follows:

> Little soul, winsome and wayward,
>> now my body's house guest and playmate,
> say now, whither will you wander,
>> shivering, pale and uncovered,
> now the time of our game is over?

Clearly the idea lingers on. The translator was aware that the time of games would end.

In closing, I provide some thoughts by Thomas More, who was not ill at the time, but who was confronted by a distressingly short trudge up Tower Hill and who knew perfectly well what acute episode lay ahead. He wrote this to his daughter, Margaret Roper, on the day before his death: "Farewell my dear child and pray for me, / and I shall for you and all your friends / that we may merrily meet in Heaven."

I do not believe that these ideas have been lost from our society, nor that they have become unpopular. Physicians have dealt with them in the past and will inevitably continue to deal with them.

References

John Betjeman's collected poems. 1958. Comp. Earl of Birkenhead. Boston: Houghton Mifflin.

Waley, A. 1970. *Madly singing in the mountains.* New York: Walker and Company.

Chapter 7

The Changing Face of Death in Children

Diane M. Komp

> Children are waiting. They conduct a
> vigil while adult debates whirl around
> them. They are waiting for voices to be
> raised that represent their small best
> interests. Small and powerless, they need
> a champion to take up their cause.
> —Valerie Bell, *Nobody's Children*

The first part of this book describes some of the adult debates that whirl around us. Reading these stories of patients dying in hospitals without comfort or respect reminds me why I titled one of my books *A Child Shall Lead Them: Lessons in Hope from Children with Cancer* (1993). I firmly believe that those caring for adults facing death have much to learn from those deaths that we choose to call "untimely": the deaths of children.

Death has changed for children in the United States over the twenty-seven years that define my career. Doctors' and nurses' concepts of compassionate companioning of the dying—envisioned by humanists and religionists, yearned for by the sick, wished for by health care professionals if they could only learn how—are not in conflict with the academic mission of such an institution as Yale University School of Medicine.

You and I would like to believe that death does not wear a child's face, but it simply is not so. Death wears a child's face and always has. It always will. The only thing that will change with time is how many children will die, and where, and in what manner.

Every year in the United States more than fifteen thousand children die between the first and fourteenth years of life. The focus of this chapter is on deaths that can be anticipated—those in which physicians, nurses, and other health care professionals play an integral role, and for which we advise families about decisions surrounding the entire process. I will primarily reflect on deaths from the disease that throughout my career has maintained its position as the leading cause of death from disease in childhood. Even cancer sometimes wears the face of a child.

DISCLOSURE OF DIAGNOSIS, DISCLOSURE OF DEATH

Twenty-seven years ago, most children who were referred to specialized hospitals for cancer ultimately died from the disease. Disclosure of diagnosis was closely linked to discussion of death. That grim reality markedly affected the tone of the initial discussion with families about diagnosis and treatment. As I spoke with one young mother, telling her that her only child had leukemia, I thought, "There will be another conversation like this one in the future. Even if he goes into remission, there will be a relapse. This child will surely die." Two years later he relapsed. Five years after that conversation, the child died from leukemia.

Contrast this story with our experience today. Although cancer remains the leading cause of death from disease in childhood, the number of such deaths of children has dropped by sixty-seven percent during my career alone. Although cancer remains identified with death in the popular mind, there is reasonable hope for the majority of parents that their own child will outlive that diagnosis.

Today, doctors communicate this "reasonable hope" in initial discussions with parents; at the same time, we tell them that their child may die from this particular disease. Thus, disclosure of the diagnosis of cancer is no longer automatically linked with death. Within our same technology resides the power to harm and the power to heal. Life and death coexist, side by side.

Consider the case of a child who was diagnosed at age three with leukemia but who has relapsed and is facing death at age eight. She knew the words "leukemia" and "cancer" from that early age, but her fears were not linked to the name of a disease. She understood fear in the faces of her parents and her separation from them. Cancer was simply the reason she came to the hospital, took medication, and received special attention from her family in particular and from society at large. For her, "cancer" was a word, not a sentence.

Children with cancer don't first learn about cancer as the cause of someone else's death. They learn about it as a part of their own life. Although there is much written about children's understanding of death from a developmental, age-related point of view (Hostler 1978, 1–25), these stages of understanding cannot be freely applied to children who have grown up with a life-threatening illness as part of their lives. They do not hear baby talk at their hospitals; they list adults among their closest friends. They train their caregivers to find the words that frame a merciful version of the truth.

SPIRITUAL CARE

Other chapters will specifically address the importance of religious traditions in the care of the dying. Hospital chaplain staff and community clergy representing the family are willing resources to assist the family. This, however, does not exempt health care professionals from knowing enough about our patients' belief systems to treat them with respect.

Helpful questions to ask while taking a medical history are if and how faith and belief assist the patient and family in facing illness. We will learn such things as the orthodox Jewish attitude toward autopsy, Jehovah's Witnesses' beliefs about blood transfusion, and much more, if we will just listen.

The concept that death is "always irreversible," based on knowledge gained only by scientific methods, may conflict with firmly held religious beliefs of our patients such as a bodily resurrection, reincarnation, or an immortal soul. Although scientists hear the question "Why me?" as an epidemiological, etiological one, many families frame their "why's" in a spiritual context. The role of health care professionals is not to undermine beliefs that are a source of comfort, support, and hope to their patients but to work as best we can with families and humbly accompany them on their painful journey.

In his "Peanuts" cartoons, Charles Schulz often uses children to express the cares and concerns of the adult world. "I wonder if I'm dying?" asked Charlie Brown, and then, "I wonder if they'd tell me if I were dying?" We might question whether these thoughts truly belong to a child, but surely the feelings expressed rightfully belong to this child character. Later, Charlie Brown tells us the source of his fear. "First I was surrounded by doctors and nurses. Now everybody's gone."

Children are as expert as adults in reading the faces of their doctors and nurses. But they are more expert than adults in tending to important relationships. And they have high (but reasonable) expectations from those whose companionship they value. The major fears children with cancer express about death are of separation and isolation. Separation and isolation while they are in the valley of the shadow of death are preventable disorders.

OPEN DISCUSSION OF DEATH

A quarter century ago, few pediatric oncologists advocated open discussion of death with children. In the past, doctors avoided open discussion of death with all patients. But we stand today on the "other side of Kübler-Ross."[1] There are some assumptions garnered from adult experience that have guided professional wisdom about dying children in recent years.

We assume that open discussion is better than failure to discuss. We also assume that when children are dying they will want to talk about their deaths. A 1993 study confirms a dramatic shift in professional opinion.

Goldman and Christie report that 100 percent of their team members favored open discussion of death with children dying with cancer. What this high vote of confidence does not reveal is how often that advocacy is translated into actual practice.

Their data came from interviews of families after the death of the child. In contrast to the universal approval of openness, the approach of death was mutually acknowledged by the minority of children and parents—a mere 19 percent. In 29 percent of cases, parents believed that the child died without being aware that he was dying. Furthermore, 23 percent of these parents did not know what their child knew about death. Another 23 percent assumed that the child knew but did not wish to discuss it. Six percent of parents even blocked open discussion of death with their child.

So if health care professionals think that there should be open discussion and parents don't often do it, who should tell a child about impending death? I've asked this question of parents in bereavement groups across the country. Unless we maintain contact with families after death, we will not learn what they carried away from the experience. Let me summarize my experiences with parents whose children knew about their deaths.

Those parents whose children learned of relapse or death without the parents present carried this as an "unforgivable" failure of the staff. Their anger persisted for years after the child's death. When doctors or nurses were caught unawares by a direct question from the child and communicated their responses to the parents, they had no difficulty. But parents resented intrusion of health care professionals into areas that they considered parental prerogative. The best experiences were those where doctors and nurses advised parents about how to listen to their own children. The following case illustrates this point.

When Tony relapsed, I told his parents not only about the medical details of clinical death, but advised them to listen to their child. Some weeks later, his mother reported that, out of the blue, Tony said: "He wants me."

His mother was frightened but found the courage to ask him, "Do you mean God?" When Tony nodded, his mother asked when God spoke to him.

"He speaks to me when I pray," her fifteen-year-old son answered.

"What do you mean, 'when you pray'?" This did not fit in with the family's manner of praying.

"I start praying," the boy said, "and then I listen."

A frightened mother listened carefully to her son. Some weeks later, he said, "I don't want to die yet. Gerry [his youngest brother] is only three and is not old enough to understand. I've been able to talk to each of my other brothers to prepare them and they'll be okay. I can leave a letter for Gerry but it's not the same. If I could live just one more year, I could explain it to him myself and he will understand. Three is just too young."

I explained to the mother that it was just not medically possible for him to survive that additional year. Tony lived for exactly one year after that prayer on behalf of his little brother (Komp 1992). Eight years later, his parents and brothers remember his brave and perfect gift to those who survived.

What of those families for whom disclosures by well-intentioned health care professionals have wounded more than informed? One mother re-counted the indescribable pain she felt when a doctor took her son aside and told him of his relapse without his parents present, informing him that there was no treatment to offer. She returned to the floor to find her son weeping.

But something good came out of the experience. It came from her son's words to her when he dried his tears. "You are the best mother I could ever have hoped for. You have taken such good care of me. After I die, I want you to study to be a nurse. You can be such a great help to other kids like me." This wise, dying child gave a great, great legacy to children with cancer who will follow him.

DEATH AT HOME

Let me go on to two other assumptions that doctors make. We assume that the more knowledgeable a family is, the more accepting they will be of the futility of treatment. Furthermore we assume that death at home is preferred by children and parents to death in the hospital.

I reviewed our own institutional experience of deaths of children with blood conditions and cancer over a two-and-a-half-year period. I per-formed a related study fifteen years ago and observed that with support from the staff, 50 percent of children with leukemia could be cared for terminally in their own homes (Komp and Fortunato, 1978). But current data from the Department of Pediatrics at Yale University School of Medi-cine show that this figure has not improved. Only one-third of our children with cancer who die today die at home.

Given the type of institution we work in, two questions come to mind: Does the active pursuit of clinical research by the treating physicians bias them against simpler palliative care? Second, does the interposition of younger physicians in training influence these choices?

Three cohorts of patients were identified: (1) those whose primary hema-tologist-oncologist was a full-time faculty member, (2) those whose pri-mary hematologist-oncologist was a postdoctoral fellow under the supervision of a full-time faculty member, and (3) those whose primary hematolo-gist-oncologist was a private practitioner. The patients came to the same hospital and shared the same nurses, social workers, psychologists, psychiatrists, and chaplain staff.

Small numbers do not permit statistical conclusions, simply observations of trends with these thirty-six deaths. Forty-four percent of the faculty patients died at home, in comparison to 36 percent of patients cared for by trainees and none of the private patients during the study period. Thus, these trends suggest that youthfulness of physicians, academic orientation of attending physicians, and participation in clinical research protocols for cancer treatment need not stand in the way of, or bias against, death at home.

More notable in this series is the repetition of a finding from the older study. Children who survived more than six months after diagnosis were more likely (41 percent versus 10 percent) to die at home than those who died less than six months after diagnosis. The single death at home in the early death group was a child with Down's syndrome whose family had already considered these issues and options before the diagnosis of leukemia. Thus, anticipation of death and time for preparation continue to outweigh the specifics of disease manifestations, physician preferences, and nursing care requirements.

Death at home is appropriate only when the option is acceptable to patients and their families. The following case illustrates this problem.

As Jim's death approached, the postdoctoral fellow supervising his case tried to arrange for him to die at home. For the patient, this was a frightening consideration, even though his young doctor, with whom he had a warm personal relationship, planned to make house calls and maintain close contact. Jim expressed his fear of bleeding to death and his fear of death. The postdoctoral fellow asked me to talk to Jim and his mother.

In discussing his fears, Jim recalled times during his illness when he was alone in the house while his widowed mother worked to maintain his health insurance. Jim was one of our growing group of "latchkey kids" with cancer. He expressed guilt that his mother had to work so hard to provide for him. He worried about what would happen to her after his death.

With his permission, I shared these concerns with his mother. She understood that her son needed her permission to die. I suggested that she offer him concrete evidence of why she knew she would be okay after his death. This conversation of mother and son freed Jim from his fear of death, and he died peacefully in the hospital two days later.

AUTOPSIES

Autopsy practices provide us with a way to examine further how medical opinions about circumstances surrounding death of children differ from a layperson's point of view. In the past, it was customary for physicians to ask parents of most if not all children who died for permission to perform an autopsy. Nationally, there has been a decline in autopsies, particularly in children. Newer imaging and laboratory tests have given physicians other means for examining without invading. But there remains a wide gap between clinical and anatomic diagnosis (Di Furia et al., 1991). In some cases, knowledge of the correct diagnosis would have made a difference in the outcome of the case.

A review of deaths of children cared for by the same Yale–New Haven Hospital doctors from 1990 to 1992 reveals an overall autopsy rate of 17 percent. Of interest are the practices of managing physicians in requesting autopsies and the success in achieving parental agreement. Academic physicians and younger physicians were not more aggressive in seeking autopsies than private practitioners who were not participating in clinical research trials. None of these groups, however, was very successful in receiving permission for autopsy. There was an overall refusal rate of 68 percent, with only thirteen out of the nineteen requested autopsies actually performed.

When examining the pursuit of autopsy in relationship to time of death after diagnosis, we noted that physicians sought autopsy most often in recently diagnosed cases (78 percent versus 44 percent). Parents, however, refused at similar rates (71 percent versus 67 percent), whether their children were recently or more distantly diagnosed.

Although the literature addresses religious reasons for refusal of autopsy and the need for sensitivity to this issue, it does not adequately examine lay opinion about autopsy. The following story of one mother illustrates the point.

Bill died in the hospital after a long illness. The attending physician was present at the child's death and asked Bill's mother's permission for autopsy. She declined, and the discussion ended there. After her son's death, however, there were times when she had questions about what might have been found at autopsy. I asked the mother what her reasons were at the time for refusal. "I thought that the reason you do an autopsy is to find out who did what wrong. I think all I knew about autopsies came from watching *Quincy* on television. The pathologist was always accusing his colleagues. When the doctor asked me about autopsy, I thought she had to ask me. I told her, 'No, that's OK. We don't want one.' What I meant was that I was satisfied with my son's care and I didn't want anyone like Quincy making trouble for the doctors who took care of my son."

Today, most doctors ask permission for autopsies so that parents can have answers to their own "what ifs." And contrary to this mother's assumption, most pediatric oncologists want to learn themselves why things do not turn out the way they had hoped and planned. Unfortunately, some pathologists believe the "Quincy myth" as well. One recent book written by a pathologist for the general public perpetuates this adversarial image of colleague against colleague (Burgess 1992).

Ideally, parents should have adequate, accurate, and timely information about autopsy procedures to dispel any popular myths and permit them to make their best decisions. The following case illustrates a more successful approach than the previous one.

Brian suffered from a mysterious, undiagnosed illness transmitted in a genetic fashion in his family. Despite extraordinary attempts to establish a diagnosis, it was apparent that he would die undiagnosed. At his parents' request, he was transferred to a smaller hospital closer to the family home so that they could also attend to the needs of their other children and their anticipatory grief. We maintained telephone contact.

One of these telephone conversations occurred a month before his death. I broached the subject of autopsy. Brian's mother admitted that it was a very frightening thing to think about and that her husband was unlikely to agree. She appreciated that the conversation was occurring before her child's death and acknowledged the value to her own family of understanding this illness. She agreed to discuss it with her husband who, as predicted, was reluctant to agree. But they also agreed to talk by telephone with a pediatric pathologist who had offered consultative services to inform them about the facts and myths about autopsy.

This consultation proved invaluable to the family in reaching their decision to agree and in facilitating cooperation between the pathology departments of the two hospitals.

AIDS IN CHILDREN

Finally, we turn to another change in the face of death in children. Death from cancer has decreased in children with time, but another important disease is doing quite the opposite.

AIDS first entered the list of top causes from death from disease for children ages one to fourteen years with the 1987 listing. HIV is now the fifth leading cause of death in this age group, and in some American cities it is already the major cause of death from disease in childhood, overshadowing cancer.

By the end of 1991, an estimated 18,500 children and adolescents in this country were orphaned by the disease. Many of these children will need someone else to love them even as they face their own deaths. Unless the tide of the epidemic is turned, that figure will increase to 82,000 children and adolescents bereft of their mothers by this disease by the turn of the century (Michaels and Levine 1992). Many of these children will, in turn, die from the same dreadful disease that orphaned them.

In contrast to children with cancer, children with AIDS who learn about the disease as part of their life are likely to experience it as the cause of death of someone close to them. Few children with AIDS are told directly of their diagnosis. Despite this nondisclosure, many of the older children suspect. Hospitalized children with AIDS may seek information from their medical caregivers that was not provided by their families.

For these families, disclosure of the diagnosis not only unveils a bleak prognosis; it also unmasks the secrets and despair of other family members and exposes them to possible loss of housing and social shunning. But, like other dying children, children with AIDS know in their bodies when death is near.

Tanya was HIV-infected at birth and enjoyed good health for most of her seven years until she developed a malignancy. She and her family continued to do their best to emphasize the quality of the life she had. One day she told her family, "I need to pack a suitcase. I'm not sure if it's for the emergency room or heaven." She didn't seem critically ill, but she came to the emergency room and was admitted to the hospital. She had respiratory decompensation shortly thereafter and was transferred to the intensive care unit. Two days after admission, unexpectedly, she ate her breakfast, lay back, and died.

In her book *Nobody's Children* (1989), Valerie Bell warns us that it is hard to love somebody else's child. And yet we must if in the face of these new untimely deaths our society is to survive and we are to remain human. AIDS seems determined to teach us all what fully human means.

THE FAMILY OF THE DYING CHILD

In times past, the death of a child was part of a family's life, not a medical event. There were no medical figures or equipment to intrude on the family's grief. Today, we as health care professionals are challenged by the humane deaths of these past times. We must learn how to provide support for families without suggesting that for a good death to happen we have to run the show. We must provide the support needed, but not take center stage.

The story of a modern child makes an appropriate summary statement. This thirteen-year-old boy's parents wanted to know the right thing to say to help their son find peace in his death. I suggested that we listen to their son to find the cues they needed. His mother introduced me, and Scotty was intrigued.

"I hear that you write books," he said to me. "So, what do you write about?"

"I talk to kids like you," I said, "and I write their stories. I'm just the secretary. Kids like you have taught me that I don't have all the answers and I need some good teachers." He smiled, pleased that I knew my place in the world.

"You know," he said, measuring his labored breaths, planning the lesson he had in mind. "Not everything in science is true. And not everything in religion is true either."

"What is it in science that you think isn't true?" I asked him.

"Well, take that 'big bang' theory. It doesn't seem very logical to me. When I look at the world, I can't believe that it happened by accident. I could be wrong, but it doesn't seem to make a lot of sense."

"And what is it about religion that you don't think is true?" I pressed.

"Well, take David and Goliath."

"What about David and Goliath?" I was curious. I never before met a kid who had trouble with David and Goliath.

"Goliath couldn't have been eight foot three tall," he said. "There's nobody that tall."

"I've seen some pretty tall basketball players," I offered.

"Not that tall," he shook his head, dismissing my suggestion.

"There's a pituitary condition where people make too much growth hormone," I tried again.

"None. Nobody that tall. But you know, it's not the details that matter. It's the moral of the story. Do you know what the moral of the story is?"

The moral of both stories is that a little kid can prevail against something that is unbelievably big. In the end, it was Scotty's wisdom that guided his parents in exercising their own. My wish for all who care about and for the dying is that somewhere in your own life there will be at least one little child to lead you.

Note

1. For more on Elisabeth Kübler-Ross, see her *On Death and Dying* (1969).

References

Bell, V. 1989. *Nobody's children.* Dallas: Word Books.
Burgess, S. B. 1992. *Understanding the autopsy.* Burnsville, N.C.: Celo Valley Books. Reprinted in *New England Journal of Medicine* 330 (1994): 1165–66.

Di Furia, L., A. Piga, S. Marmili, et al. 1991. The value of necropsy in oncology. *European Journal of Cancer* 27: 559–61.

Goldman, A., and D. Christie. 1993. Children with cancer talk about their own deaths. *Pediatric Hematology/Oncology* 10: 223–31.

Hostler, S. 1978. The development of the child's concept of death. In *The child and death,* ed. D. J. Sahler. St. Louis, Mo.: C. V. Mosby.

Komp, D. M. 1992. *A window to heaven: When children see life in death.* Grand Rapids, Mich.: Zondervan.

Komp, D. M. 1993. *A child shall lead them: Lessons in hope from children with cancer.* Grand Rapids, Mich.: Zondervan.

Komp, D. M., and R. P. Fortunato. 1978. Childhood leukemia: Perspectives 1978. *Virginia Medical Monthly* 105: 622.

Kübler-Ross, E. 1969. *On death and dying.* New York: Macmillan.

Michaels, D., and C. Levine. 1992. Estimate of the number of motherless youth orphaned by AIDS in the United States. *Journal of the American Medical Association* 268: 3456.

Chapter 8

When Children Mourn a Loved One

Morris A. Wessel

Twenty-five years ago, Florence Wald invited me to join a few colleagues who met monthly to study the experiences of patients and families in the terminal phase of life. For me, these meetings were an oasis in a vast medical institution where computers, monitoring devices, and the increasing specialization of medical care made it difficult for patients to live fully and with dignity to the end.

Very quickly, despite our diverse professional and religious backgrounds, we were drawn together by a common reverence for human life. We found satisfaction in sharing thoughts, anxieties, concerns, and anguish. I soon became challenged to consider ways in which I as a primary pediatrician might enhance the capacity of parents and children to deal with losses of loved ones.

At the outset of my pediatric practice in 1951, I had decided to encourage expectant parents to arrange for a conference during the last trimester of pregnancy. As I inquired about details of a family's medical history, I discovered that many expectant parents had suffered the loss of a parent during childhood. I was surprised that many men and women cried as they shared memories of their losses during the first decade of their life. Many persons recalled having been sent to neighbors or to school at the time of a family member's funeral. A common memory was described in this manner: "When I returned home, there were lots of people around. Everyone was silent and weeping. No one had time for me. I didn't know what to do with myself. All I remember is that the person I loved had disappeared and I never saw her again."

This removal of children from the funeral service was intended to spare them the agony of participating. I learned, however, that this practice denied children the support of this important ritual, one which adults consider so important for themselves. I was fortunate at this time to read *A*

Child's Parent Dies (Furman 1974), a study of young children who had suffered the loss of a parent during their preschool years. This book helped me guide parents who sought my advice for how to help children who were grappling with the loss of loved ones.

I now am convinced that, difficult as it may seem, it is important to offer children five years and older the opportunity to participate in a funeral or memorial service. I usually suggest that a close family friend accompany the children because the immediate family members are often preoccupied with their own grieving and have little energy to comfort a child.

As children struggle to accept the reality of the loss, they may ask whether the deceased will return for a birthday or an important family holiday. If a child has attended the service, one can simply say: "You remember we said good-bye at the funeral. I too miss her very much. We will have to remember all those happy times when she was with us."

Adapting to a significant loss is never an easy task. The manner in which a child is supported at this tragic moment often determines whether it remains an overwhelming, unmasterable burden interfering seriously with his development or a stress that the child copes with and integrates into his personality as he matures. Mourning is a sad process for children as well as adults. It is important that adults who nurture children support and comfort them as they grieve and mourn in their own way over time. The goal is not to prevent sadness in children, but rather to comfort and support them in their sadness.

Children may ask what happens to persons when they die. I suggest that depending on their own religious beliefs parents answer the question honestly and simply by stating, for example: "I like to believe that Grandpa is in some place far away called Heaven, where there is no suffering."

If such a conceptualization is foreign to the beliefs of the family member, they may want to comment: "I am not certain what I believe. I do know that many people believe that a person who dies rests in a far away place called Heaven." It is important to mention this concept so that a child will understand comments by friends who may discuss their own religious convictions of a life hereafter.

Parents are often upset at their tendency to cry as children ask poignant questions. I believe that this is not a harmful experience. Children observing an adult in tears often feel it gives them permission to express their sad feelings in a similar fashion. A warm hug as a parent and child cry allows them to express their sadness together.

A child who has experienced a recent loss is easily frightened when other family members are away, fearing that they too might disappear forever. I advise parents and other nurturers to inform a child where they are going and when they will return. They should telephone if there is any delay in returning home.

Children suffering a loss may regress to immature behavior. They may become anxious at bedtime and fearful about leaving home. They may be restless, whiny, and find it difficult to involve themselves in usual activities. They may return to outgrown bowel habits. Poor school performance is also common during bereavement. I suggest that parents notify a child's teacher of the sad events so that he or she can be understanding when a child behaves in an unusual manner.

The death of a parent or other beloved person during adolescence has unique effects because of the development that occurs during this phase of life. At one moment, healthy adolescents are independent, determined to make their own way in the world. At other times, particularly after a stressful period, adolescents may revert to a less mature stage, seeking parental care, sympathy, and advice. Such fluctuations between independence and dependence are normal at this age. The usual family constellation with two parents allows the adolescent to break away gradually on a trial basis and to thrive on activity outside the family setting. Yet during phases of intense independence, when adolescents may be critical of parents, there still remains the comforting option to return home and be taken care of as in former years. The death of a parent eliminates this option.

A bereaved child or adolescent dreads any illness. A call from a family who has experienced a significant loss merits prompt attention. A careful examination usually rules out any serious disease. One can reassure that exhaustion, headaches, poor appetite, abdominal discomfort, and disturbed sleep are experienced commonly during bereavement. However, serious illnesses do occur among bereaved children. Complaints at this stressful moment may represent symptoms of malabsorption syndrome, cardiac arrhythmia, asthma, peptic ulcer, or inflammatory bowel disease. Lowered resistance to viral infections is also common during this period of stress.

There is one other important aspect of serving families who have experienced a recent loss. I always ask parents how they are feeling. The usual response is a noncommittal "all right." Bereaving adults often report that friends and relatives attempt to urge them to return to full activity long before they have had time to deal with their recent loss. Colin Murray Parkes, in his *Bereavement: Studies of Grief in Adult Life* (1972) helped me understand the natural history of this experience. I mention to the grieving persons that bereavement is a long and painful process. I also tell them that in the Jewish tradition, one expects it to take at least a year after a loss before an individual can begin to function with reasonable normalcy. Many parents in my practice expressed many months later their appreciation for my mentioning the human need to grieve and mourn over time.

References

Furman, E. 1974. *A child's parent dies: Studies in childhood bereavement*. New Haven, Conn.: Yale University Press.
Parkes, C. 1972. *Bereavement: Studies of grief in adult life*. New York: International Universities Press.

Chapter 9

The Emergence of Hospice Care in the United States

Florence S. Wald

The concept of hospice care for terminally ill patients came to the United States in 1963. The first hospice home care services were offered in the greater New Haven area in 1974. By 1994 there were two thousand hospices nationwide.

What accounts for such widespread rapid growth? Hospice was a radical departure from technologic medicine. When Dr. Cicely Saunders brought her ideas of hospice from England, one of her stops in 1963 was Yale University Medical Center. Bernard Lytton, then head of the Urology Department, asked her to tell the medical students about her approach to patients with far advanced cancer. She told them how suffering could be eased, leaving patients and families available to attend to their relationships in the closing chapter of life of one of their members. Her approach began with a careful assessment of the patient from every standpoint—medical, psychological, spiritual, social, and economic—to uncover what patients wanted for themselves. Her comprehensive knowledge of drugs and their interactions opened a new avenue to comfort while leaving the patient as alert as possible until the end. Her knowledge had a broad base, for she had been educated as a nurse, an almoner, and a physician. She added two years of experience in clinical trials of palliative care in St. Joseph's Hospice in London before she set off on her long-planned dream, a clinical setting of her own making.

Yale's third-year medical students gave Saunders a standing ovation. She also made an indelible impression on me, for until then I had thought nurses were the only people troubled by how a terminal illness was treated. In the Yale University Nursing School, where I was dean, faculty and students had found themselves at cross purposes with doctors when patients asked questions about their illness. Doctors evaded questions about outcome and progress, especially those about treatments that failed to improve the patient's health and about a life coming to a close. At best, nurses were rebuffed; at worst, they were barred from care. Their most troubling questions were "Is the treatment working?" "Will you help me ask the doctor?" and "How long will it be?"

Ida Orlando, then a member of the nursing school faculty, urged students and colleagues to encourage patients to express their thoughts and feelings about the illness and proposed treatment (Orlando 1961). In clinical studies of women in labor and of patients facing surgery, symptoms such as nausea, pain, or tension diminished in those who expressed their concerns beforehand and had support to count on. Controlled experimental studies showed the difference. Putting this approach into practice was our problem.

While much has been learned about stress in the past twenty years, in the early sixties little had been published or accepted in practice. Yet we were seeing its effects and just learning to study it systematically.

Our other pain was watching the never-ending intensive treatment carried to the bitter end as patients suffered and became more helpless. When Saunders visited Yale, pediatrician Ray Duff and sociologist August Hollingshead were engaged in a descriptive study of the communications patients and families had with caregivers in hospitals. But it wasn't until their book *Sickness and Society* was published in 1968 that they described what happened when patients were dying. They wrote:

> A patient who was terminally ill created crises in human relations for those who were caring for him. One dilemma arose from the fact that not every member of the group involved—the sick person, the spouse, the responsible physician, nurses, and other family members—realized the illness was a fatal one. It may have been in the interests of some persons to mislead other members of the group. Evasions, silences, half-truths, and deliberate lies then became elements in the social realities that tied the group together and in turn influenced the communications of one person with another. A second dilemma arose from the lack of explicit norms in our culture to guide the day-to-day relations of the group as death approached. A third revolved around the uncertainty of when death would occur.

A VISION FOR CHANGE

Saunders's vision of patient and family in the foreground and treatment in the background and her conviction that listening was an essential act took hold of me. I wondered: could this approach survive in a medical center such as ours? My experience as a dean had taught me how much effort was needed to revamp curriculums, develop new services, or change long-accepted practice.

Fortunately, the sixties were a time when change happened in many institutions. The church and its ministers led freedom marches to protest inequality of the races. New ways to express democratic values came with the way and degree in which congregant members participated in rituals. Thinking about work and lifestyle in terms of one's values encouraged Christians to express themselves as followers of Christ. The changes in Catholic churches were most noticeable. Where the altar was placed, who took part in the service, the language spoken, and even the establishment of home churches evidenced democratization and opened communication between clergy and parish.

At universities, colleges, and schools, protests against the war in Vietnam were expressed for the most part without violence, but were highly visible. A part in governance and freedom of speech were the demands. Law was soon involved, as rules and regulations interfaced with rights and responsibilities of individuals and institutions.

It was in this atmosphere that patients' rights and informed consent came to the surface. Doctors, nurses, and even patients sought out ethicists and lawyers to examine their practices and policies. In addition, the rise of the women's movement gave promise that the gender barrier between doctors (predominantly men) and nurses (predominantly women) would be lowered—that doctors would hear what nurses said and nurses would challenge doctors. The health care hierarchy was shaken. Nurses became more capable of expressing themselves and began to expect recognition.

It was a propitious time for health care reforms, a time for change. Examining professional roles and responsibilities made caregivers aware of their own spiritual values whether religious, secular, or both. In this context new questions arose.

How much had the ability of medicine to transform pathology in the human body caused medicine to overlook the cost in human suffering and in dollars? How much had nursing conformed to the role of handmaiden to doctors instead of aid to the patient? Where was the balance between finite life of the body and infinite meaning of life? An interdisciplinary minority was coalescing, nationwide and worldwide, to bond health and human values.

Against this background of ethical foment and beginning change, interest in hospice grew. During her next visit in 1966, Cicely Saunders made medical rounds in various departments and met the new director of religious ministry, Edward Dobihal. Her visit ended with a workshop of thirty professionals from different disciplines, some from the medical center and others from a distance. Elisabeth Kübler-Ross (University of Chicago) and Colin Murray Parkes (University of London) later would be at the forefront of the death and dying movement, but at that time all felt they were isolated professionals reaching out to one another. Over the next four years, hundreds and sometimes more than a thousand people would come to hear Saunders and Kübler-Ross speak in various cities around the country. Most audiences comprised nurses, clergy, and social workers; later doctors came too. Kübler-Ross and Saunders were both charismatic but quite different. Elisabeth Kübler-Ross was zealous: she inspired caregivers to be unafraid, to reach out to dying patients, and to be guided by feelings—gut feelings—and intuition. She had boundless energy. When the department of psychiatry of the University of Chicago failed to renew her appointment, she took to the road as an independent lecturer and consultant. So began her odyssey, first national and then international. Her lectures were attended by thousands; her workshops lasted for days, many of them well into the night. Ultimately she built a center of her own, Shanti Nilaya. Soon her audiences included patients and families. Of professionals, nurses were the ones who appreciated her most. Rather than conforming her teaching and practice to academic and professional rules and regulations, Kübler-Ross created her own institution, which flourished for twenty-five years. Using intuition and incorporating women's ways of knowing were her greatest gifts. Her concept of life after death earned her detractors.

Cicely Saunders's career was more traditional. Inspired as early as 1947 to ease the suffering of cancer patients, she had become nurse, almoner, and physician. She knew what the medical establishment expected and regulatory agencies prescribed. She struck a balance between accepted practice and new ideas. Because her spiritual foundation was profoundly in the Anglican Church, she kept its church leaders informed of and involved in her plans for St. Christopher's. She cultivated ties to the medical establishment as well; she was a member of the Royal College of Physicians.

Having gone through all the steps of planning and building St. Christopher's, she became our mentor in each stage of creating the Connecticut Hospice. The process began in 1969. I returned from a month's internship at St. Christopher's Hospice in London and quickly found Dr. Morris Wessel and the Rev. Dobihal to join what was to become an interdisciplinary team. Ira Goldenberg, an oncologic surgeon, became the principal physician. In a short time, two Catholic priests and a Lutheran minister (Fathers Don McNeil and Robert Canney and Pastor Fred Auman) and finally a second nurse, Katherine L. Klaus, were added as members.

CHANGE FROM WITHIN

The strategy at Yale was to provide a service to the institution we knew, with all its strengths and weaknesses. We didn't ask for beds; they were always difficult to get. We asked those in charge of specific units to allow us to be the caregivers for terminally ill patients. Two nurses, Katherine Klaus and I, gave nursing care and recorded acts, conversations, thoughts, and feelings in our diaries as participant-observers. Patients and their families were told that we were keeping diaries about their care that would ultimately be published without their identities being disclosed. In return, we gave them care when and where it was needed in the hospital, home, or nursing home. We thought that working within the existing setting in that way would illuminate what components of care were missing and which were already provided. Yale University Schools of Nursing and Medicine sponsored the two-year project; the Nursing Division of the United States Public Health Service and the American Nurses Foundation provided the funds.

Helplessness was the condition patients found most difficult. All of us found living with uncertainty our greatest challenge. "How long?" "What's coming next?" "Am I slipping?" and "Will the money last?" were frequent questions.

The length of the terminal phase was unpredictable. Twenty patients were expected to die within three months; of these, one lived eight months and three lived more than a year. Three patients who seemed stable died unexpectedly within twenty-four hours. Five patients deemed terminal chose aggressive treatment almost until the end. There was no certain answer to "How long?" But our contract with them—to give care and be with them at home, hospital, or nursing home—gave them the assurance we would be there when they needed us.

"What's coming next?" had different connotations. "Next" might mean in the next hour; during the program for the day; or beyond the time when present therapy is abandoned. The question might also be a way of asking what the options are if the present treatment fails, or what happens when this life ends. The nurse who is alert to how patients are experiencing the situation has more of an opportunity to seize the moment, to find out what the patients want for themselves today, in a while, or in a crisis. It took courage to follow this path. The process led to a review of life, a search for meaning or painful secrets patients needed to share. The patients' search for their spiritual roots, religious or secular, brought us to strange territory. It also took time and flexibility—willingness to shift priorities.

The question "Am I slipping?" was hard, too. Losing an ability, a pound, or strength could seem like a start down a slippery slope. We learned that there were ups and downs, sometimes roller coaster changes, and that there were plateaus. Our experience made us look at our plan of care for omission or commission.

In the beginning it was frustrating to see how little time hospital staff spent with patients and how infrequently they followed patients' problems to solutions. Morris Wessel helped us see the reasons for differences. Dying patients need time and human presence. Curable patients need quick action and technology. The pacing is different, and caregivers look for different cues.

Dr. Goldenberg, as had been predicted by his medical colleagues, kept in touch with patients and families whether there was improvement or decline. We saw how patients' faces lit up when he entered the room. One said, "All he has to do is walk in the room and I feel better!" I soon observed the overlapping turf of doctors and nurses and the doctor's need to be the primary, closest caregiver. Some staff nurses envied us the time and peace we had to be with patients, to hear them out, talk, and even sit in silence without the constant call to do. They lifted a disapproving eyebrow when they saw family members giving the care while Kathy or I fetched the needed linen or equipment as if we were nurses' aides. They didn't see how much the family gained by giving care.

Pharmacologic relief of symptoms—using morphine, not Demerol; Benadryl for anxiety; analgesics in anticipation rather than when the pain was unbearable—never gained acceptance by hospital nurses or physicians. Now, twenty-five years later, pain management is far better understood and practiced. Then it was in hot dispute.

Finally, the concern "Will the money last?" seems closely connected with the sense of helplessness. None of the twenty-two patients ended up in debt, but all that the families had was depleted. One patient's husband had a heart attack and died before she did. At last I understood why patients felt guilty seeing how hard the illness was on their families.

Good times, on a small scale or large, were a boost. A change in setting, hospital to home, brought a sense of freedom. When symptoms were out of control, family relations became tangled, or when we felt unsure of ourselves, however, the hospital felt safer than home. An open door, a change of heart or mind were needed options. Pacing was important. One patient said she could tell what kind of a day it would be when she got out of bed and put her slippers on. She planned her day accordingly. The more energetic the patients, the more accustomed they were to a vigorous life, the harder it was for them to no longer be able to count on a usual day. The nurses' pace needed slowing, too. It was not just a matter of sitting quietly with the patient, but of learning the uses of silence—to turn over an idea and digest a thought before expressing it. Insights come in silence.

Taking a spring drive over back roads with a patient, a widow with three teenage sons, gave us the privacy we needed to think how to answer her sons' questions about her illness. They had told Dr. Goldenberg they knew she was dying; she had given them false reassurance. Another patient became comatose after intensive radiation, and while her sisters and I sat with her they told me about their childhood, parents, and life in New Haven. On the third day the patient awoke. She told us a dream about a fence that enclosed a tree and four bicycles. Her sisters knew what it meant: she was worried about the size of the cemetery plot where her parents were buried—that there wouldn't be enough room. She wanted to be buried in a place where the graves of her husband and children could be near hers. At last her sisters promised to do as she asked. They said they knew she was dying, and they promised to care for her husband and children.

THE HOSPICE MOVEMENT QUICKENS

By the time our study ended in 1971, professionals in a wide sweep across North America had become inspired by Kübler-Ross and by Saunders to take a first step toward care for the terminally ill. The interest and enthusiasm of the professionals was matched by that of the public. As we began the planning of a hospice for the greater New Haven area, volunteers clamored to help with fund-raising, publicity, office chores, and later, inpatient care. The surge and interest were unstoppable.

The interdisciplinary team that had worked together since 1969 at Yale (Auman, Canney, Dobihal, Goldenberg, Klaus, Wald, and Wessel) became founders along with Henry Wald (a health facility planner) and incorporated the hospice as an independent, not-for-profit institution.

The home care services of our hospice began in 1974, and the in-patient facility was built and opened in 1980. The components of hospice care emerged from clinical experience and a vast amount of writing, research, and teaching. The forms of hospice services vary from community to community, region to region, state to state, and nation to nation. A particular form was usually molded by the services a community already had, so that some hospices sprang from existing visiting nurse agencies, and some hospitals gave over a wing, or part of one, where the terminally ill were cared for by nurses and doctors whose goal was palliative care. Some hospitals provided a palliative team to be aides, consultants, and advisors to the hospital staff who care for the terminally ill. There are also a few free-standing hospices.

While the forms are different among hospice programs, the assumptions, principles, and standards of care are not. The International Work Group on Death, Dying, and Bereavement, founded in 1974, set down some initial assumptions and principles, and in the United States the National Hospice Organization sets current standards. Under these guidelines, chaplains, doctors, nurses, and social workers compose the interdisciplinary team. Paid staff share the work with volunteers.

The patient has not only a physiologic dimension but also social and spiritual dimensions. Pain, for example, comes not only from the changes in the body organs and systems but also from spiritual needs or from entanglements in social relationships. It is not only the patient who needs help, but also those left behind—the family and friends.

Care of survivors has taught much about one's process of letting go, readiness to cease grieving, and recovery from loss. The practice of including the family in care and for care has meant that more members of society are witnessing death and learning how to help in the process. Fear, we found, comes from misconceptions and not knowing how to help.

Hospice care does not turn its back on traditional intensive treatments of disease; it offers an alternative. Many hospice workers see that an open system of care has not yet been achieved. The International Work Group on Death, Dying, and Bereavement (Corr et al. 1994) makes this intent clear.

> Patients with life-threatening illnesses, including progressive malignancies, need appropriate therapy and treatment throughout the course of illness. At one stage, therapy is directed toward assessment and intervention in order to control and/or to cure such illness and alleviate associated symptoms. For some persons, however, the time comes when cure and remission are beyond current medical expertise. It is then that the intervention must shift to what is now often termed "Palliative treatment," which is designed to control pain in the broadest sense and provide personal support for patients and family during the terminal phase of illness. In general, palliative care requires limited use of apparatus and technology, extensive personal care, and an ordering of the physical and social environment to be therapeutic in itself.

RECOGNITION AND REENTRY

Whom do hospices serve? It varies. Most hospice patients have far advanced cancer. When the AIDS epidemic surfaced in 1982, most hospices admitted AIDS patients, and new hospices only for AIDS patients were created. There is now a trend to serve patients with other advanced degenerative diseases, such as chronic heart disease and kidney failure, to integrate patients in a less advanced stage of illness whose treatment is on the borderline between intensive treatment and palliation.

The ebb and flow of disease is unpredictable, yet patients should have options at all stages of their illness. A patient may come in very frail and failing rapidly but will improve when underlying causes—panic, diabetic coma, impacted bowel, disintegrating family relations, tumor pressing on a vital organ—are treated with intensive personal care or comfort measures. Once revived, the patient may return home. Licensure determines how long a patient can have a bed; reimbursement is set by public and private insurance. The patient who hits a plateau can be in limbo. The original goal—no limit on a patient's length of stay—is not assured. Further, Medicare stipulates that a patient must choose intensive treatment or hospice care. If the choice is hospice care, the patient is expected to relinquish intensive treatment. The intended two-way street is blocked by regulations.

Licensure of a health institution and a certificate of need are given by each state. Regulations vary. Within a region, the way the network of agencies relate to one another determines how effective and efficient total care is. Hospices, unfortunately, are not always good team players. The commitment to its value system and zeal can lead to a sense of superiority in situations where humility is needed.

In this chaotic time when hospitals, government, insurance companies, and health care workers are involved in "downsizing," reassigning responsibility for patient care, and forming new alliances and vigorous competition for who will manage care, it is rash to predict how hospices and palliative care will fit in the changing health care system.

I do, however, have some observations and hopes. First, doctors and hospitals are already linked with the private insurance sector. It seems clear that some but not all government subsidies will support intensive treatment of disease and continue dividing the work among medical specialties.

But a separate domain can emerge if primary care and preventive care take place in the community with family, doctors, and nurses as principal caregivers. The charge should be health maintenance during the entire life cycle and recovery from illness. Each stage of life would be addressed, beginning with antepartal care, natural childbirth, immunization and health education for children and young adults, the healing of body and mind throughout the adult years, instruction on how to live with old age, and assistance in facing the end of life.

Birthing centers, schools, health maintenance organizations, centers for the aging, and hospices could provide the services. What we need most of all are figurative and literal bridges between services that support the life cycle and the hospitals that change the course of disease.

References

Corr, C. A., J. D. Morgan, and H. Wass, eds. 1994. *Statements on death, dying and bereavement.* International Work Group on Death, Dying, and Bereavement, Kings College, London, Ontario.

Duff, R., and A. Hollingshead. 1968. *Sickness and society.* New York: Harper & Row.

Orlando, I. J. 1961. *The dynamic nurse-patient relationship: Function, process and principles.* New York: Putnam.

Chapter 10

Caring for Those Who Die in Old Age

Joanne Lynn

> The last night that she lived,
> It was a common night,
> Except the dying; this to us
> Made nature different. . . .
>
> We waited while she passed;
> It was a narrow time,
> Too jostled were our souls to speak,
> At length the notice came.
>
> She mentioned, and forgot;
> Then lightly as a reed
> Bent to the water, shivered scarce,
> Consented, and was dead.
>
> And we, we placed the hair,
> And drew the head erect;
> And then an awful leisure was,
> Our faith to regulate—
> —Emily Dickinson

These are the kinds of passings that I remember most: "shivered scarce, consented, and was dead." Nothing terribly dramatic, just a passing on. What is dying like, now that we have so much treatment to offer? There is much to learn. Sometimes the story the patient presents is a powerful instructor.

Here is one of the stories that I wrote for the Yale collection *Empathy and the Practice of Medicine* (Lynn 1993, 43–44):

Ask anyone who is young and healthy what it is to live well and the responses will be predictable: productivity, wealth, comfort, friends, and so on. While those things retain some value for those near death, my patients have forced me to accept much broader and more varied definitions of living well.

As a neophyte physician for a home care service, I went to see an octogenarian couple at home; Mr. Phillips with Alzheimer's-type dementia had forgotten how to swallow. This I knew how to treat. I installed a feeding tube, gave instructions, and left feeling quite good about my skills. On the next day, I received a frantic call from the home care nurse. Mrs. Phillips had called nearly incoherent and crying and the nurse wanted me to come along to reevaluate what had clearly become a crisis situation.

Mrs. Phillips met us at the door and kept repeating that she loved Bill very much and would do almost anything to help him, but that she had not been able to do what I had asked. It took a while to understand whether anything was technically difficult, or whether there had been some adverse occurrence, like aspirating or vomiting. Nothing of that sort was the problem. Mrs. Phillips finally pulled herself together enough to look at me directly and say, "I just can't tie him down to our bed." Suddenly I saw the situation from her perspective. The man with whom she had lived for sixty years and whom she had tended during nearly a decade of mental decline was not really my "problem of nutrition and hydration" but her husband, lover, and spouse. Tying him down was not a mechanical solution to the problem of keeping a feeding tube in place, but a deeply offensive abuse.

In the discussions that followed, I also realized that taking him from home in order to place a gastrostomy tube was hard to justify for his benefit and contrary to the preferences of his wife. Seeing him—and her—in their home made it easier to see the impropriety of intervention. Letting him live as well as he had been living for as long as it lasted seemed to be the best course. He died at home some two months later. The only assistance needed from the "health care system" was an aide to help with a bath most days and occasional visits from and phone calls to the home care nurse.

Consider how often we forget the humanity while we intervene to fix the physiology.

THE SEARCH FOR DATA ON DYING PATIENTS

I have been privileged in recent years to participate in some research on dying patients. The last sequential study of hospitalized dying patients in this country was done at the turn of the century. Pictured here is Sir William Osler's data collection form, filled out by a nurse within twenty-four hours of each death, sequentially, at Johns Hopkins Hospital (fig. 10.1). More than four hundred patients were studied. Osler never actually reported his findings in a journal, but he did discuss them in his talks. He found dying to be mostly quiet and he contended that helping the dying person was an important function of a physician.

It is surprising to read an older Osler textbook. At some point, everyone who cares for the dying should take one off the shelf and look at the description of any disease. Little could be done then to change the course of a disease, but much attention was given to how it affected people and to which signs indicated that things were getting worse. Osler confronted

A STUDY OF THE ACT OF DYING
Johns Hopkins Hospital

No. _____ Name _____ Hosp. No. _____ Date _____

age _____ Nationality _____ Religion. P. C. H.

Nature of disease.

Length of illness.

The act of dying:

   if sudden.

   Did respiration stop before pulse—how long?

   Coma or unconsciousness before death—how long?

   If any fear or apprehension, of what nature.

      Bodily. i.e., pain.

      Mental.

      Spiritual—remorse, etc.

   This card is not to be filled out unless done within twenty-four hours of the death of the individual.

   N. B. The object of this investigation is to ascertain the relative proportion of cases in which (1) the death is sudden: (2) accompanied by coma or unconsciousness: (3) by pain, dread or apprehension. Prof. Osler requests the intelligent co-operation of the members of the medical and nursing staff. Please note fully any other special circumstances connected with the act of dying.

Figure 10.1. Sample questionnaire from Sir William Osler's study on death and dying. Between 1900 and 1904, a total of 486 dying patients were studied at The Johns Hopkins Hospital. Courtesy of the Osler Library of the History of Medicine, McGill University, Montreal.

what happened to people as they declined and died. If you pick up an Osler text and read the chapter on diabetes, for example, you will find that it's quite openly admitted that people will die of diabetes. How they will die is described, along with how they will look and other indications that death is approaching.

Then take upon yourself the humiliating experience of picking up a standard modern American textbook. In my medical school textbook of medicine, there are over one hundred pages devoted to congestive heart failure and related subjects. The Starling curve (relating length of fiber and muscle strength) was described many times. The pharmacology of digitalis was described from multiple perspectives. But only two passages acknowledged that people die of this disease: one addressed the mortality rate after cardiac transplantation, and one gave the mortality rate from familial cardiomyopathy. Congestive heart failure is one of our most common lethal illnesses, but a modern American textbook did not acknowledge that it regularly caused death and certainly did not say what people look like as they come near that death. How do they die? How can we make dying better or worse? How can we best care for these patients? None of these issues are addressed. We need to rediscover a field that my colleague Joan Teno has named "thanatoepidemiology." We need to describe what we face as we die in order to improve it.

THE SUPPORT STUDY

I will now share some results from a forthcoming research project known as SUPPORT, for the Study to Understand Prognoses and Preferences for Outcomes and Risks of Treatment. Because this is only one study and because its data are not yet fully understood, this project places me in the position of the cartographers of old; I can only sketch the edges of the continents, the outlines of the experience of dying. But I will share with you some of this early "cartography" in the hope that you can adjust it to your own findings and maybe even be inspired to fill in some of the details that Amerigo Vespucci and I could not clearly describe.

SUPPORT enrolled every patient who came into five teaching hospitals with any of nine illnesses at an advanced stage: acute respiratory failure, congestive heart failure, multiple organ system failure with sepsis or malignancy, chronic obstructive pulmonary disease, lung cancer, cirrhosis, colon cancer, or coma. Nearly 10,000 seriously ill hospitalized patients were studied over about five years (SUPPORT 1990 and The SUPPORT Investigators, 1995). The first 4,301 patients, enrolled in a descriptive phase between 1989 and 1991, averaged sixty-three years old. The hospital mortality rate on the first admission was 27 percent. The six-month mortality was just under half.

Virtually all these patients had a fatal illness, and those who were still alive at six months remained likely to die of this illness but just hadn't died yet.

What happened near the time of death (Lynn 1995)? From interviews with surrogates, we learned that the patient was conscious about half the time and could talk within three days of death about a third of the time. Patients were in serious pain in 13 percent of the cases, had shortness of breath in 20 percent, depression in about 10 percent, and surrogates reported that the patient felt alone and isolated in 5 percent. I don't know how these descriptors look for other populations, but it is stunning that we do not have descriptors like these from many other studies.

THE SUPPORT MORTALITY MODEL

SUPPORT also developed a model to predict mortality (Knaus 1995). Most other systems to predict mortality aim to state the odds of living until a particular end point, for example, five years, one year, or leaving the hospital alive. The SUPPORT model instead estimated the patient's odds of survival for every given day over the following six months. The debate that was before Congress on the hospice benefit used the phrase "prognosis of less than six months," but no one involved in the debate ever asked what that could mean. If what you mean by "prognosis of six months" is that 1 percent or fewer survive longer, then the population you define is tiny compared to the population included if the prognosis of six months means that 50 percent are alive six months after diagnosis.

The SUPPORT study's prediction model used fourteen elements to predict this curve—a curve that was unique for each patient. The confidence intervals arose from the variance within our population and are calculated by a statistical technique known as bootstrapping. We can say with 95 percent confidence that the actual curve for our population lies within this span (see fig. 10.2).

We also have the ability to predict functional status (Wu 1995). The person whose situation is described in the figure, for example, at two months has a probability of surviving of .41, but only 5 percent will be alive and not severely dysfunctional. Severe dysfunction is defined as needing help with four or more activities of daily living or having a Sickness Impact Profile score of thirty or more. This represents the level at which a person needs constant attendance by somebody else. Such substantial disability ought to be factored into the decisions about how to manage the course to death.

DYING AT HOME

Patients in SUPPORT were asked whether they wanted to die at home. "If the doctor ever told me I probably had very little time to live, I'd rather go

Prognostic Estimates
Day 7 of Study

Disease GRP: Liver Failure with Cirrhosis.

These estimates reflect information available on 01/18/93. Future estimates will change significantly if the patient's physiologic state changes significantly. Disregard previous prognostic estimates.

Estimate of the Probability of Surviving (with confidence bars)

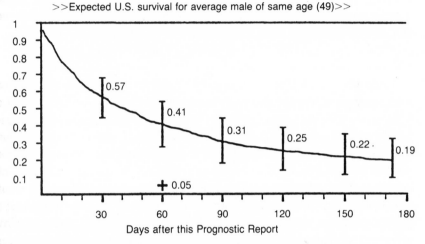

+ Probability of being alive AND not severely dysfunctional.*

Probability of not being severely dysfunctional at 2 months IF patient survives is .12 (95% CI, 0.06 to 0.25)

Figure 10.2. The SUPPORT model for time to death (Knaus 1995).

home than stay in the hospital," was one response. Of patients hospitalized with a very serious illness, 71 percent said they strongly preferred to die at home (Pritchard 1994). Of the 2,066 who died within six months, almost half died during that enrollment admission. They never got the chance to go home, though of course some might have been able to do so with adequate support. After that 914 died, and of those only 18 percent were able to die at home. Fewer than 20 percent of those who survive the initial hospitalization have the opportunity to die at home, even though over 70 percent said they very much would prefer to do so.

We could throw up our hands and say, "There's so little you could do about that. That's just the way people are. People get scared. People call 911. They end up in the hospital." However, we looked at our five sites and found that one was more than five times as likely as the others to enable patients to die at home. What does that site do differently? They have an integrated hospice and home care system. Their doctors follow their patients at home, and see it as important for people to be at home. They have the same financial incentives as everybody else, but they get people home. So some of the evidence is heartening.

Where do Americans actually die if they're not all dying in hospitals? We don't know. Death certificates are hopelessly misleading because they record where the doctor was when he or she saw the corpse, not where the death actually happened. If a funeral home brings the body by the hospital emergency room to get the death certificate signed, the death gets recorded as a hospital death. Figuring out even such simple things as where people really die is often not easy.

PAIN AND RESUSCITATION

What do we know about pain? Everybody worries about pain in cancer. In our study, however, patients have almost the same level of pain whether they die of cancer or of congestive heart failure (Desbiens 1994). Ten percent of the patients have the most severe category of pain (severe pain, most or all of the time) in all categories (except coma). Doctors don't realize facts like these. Patients with chronic obstructive pulmonary disease hurt because they are having trouble breathing or because they have tubes down their throat. The patients with congestive heart failure have ascites and the stretching hurts, or they have pain in moving and from muscle weakness. These are not just minor background conditions; they are serious and associated with the dominant illness.

How well are we handling the decision whether to try to resuscitate? Data from SUPPORT concerns very sick people in teaching hospitals that have excellent reputations. Even so, and even for patients who say they don't want resuscitation, a discussion about resuscitation is documented in the charts less than half the time (Teno 1994). These rates reflect more than simply a deficiency in charting; patients who do not want resuscitation attempted confirm this finding.

On the other hand, how are we doing with resuscitation itself? When I was in medical school during the early seventies, there was no way for a patient to escape a resuscitation attempt. One of my patients was a young woman dying from lupus whose heart finally stopped in the presence of her bishop and her family. It was a lovely deathbed scene, with tears and prayers. All that could be done for her had been done. However, the minute the monitor showed that her heart had stopped, the resuscitation team was called and she had an open-heart resuscitation effort, complete with surgically opened chest, in the presence of distraught family. There was no way at that time to prevent that practice: probably 80 to 90 percent of our patients then were subjected to a resuscitation attempt.

In SUPPORT, patients were in one of five academic teaching hospitals, lived at least forty-eight hours after admission, and had one of nine specific diseases. How many of them had a try at resuscitation as they died? Resuscitation was forgone for 84 percent of this population. Clearly, American caregivers have already learned a lot. We no longer try resuscitations on everyone who dies in a hospital.

When, however, do we write orders to forgo resuscitation? Almost all are in the last few days before death. Among persons who die, most have DNR (do not resuscitate) orders, but the median time before death is only four days. DNR orders act as last rites, not as advance planning. As the person's blood pressure is fading, we used to call the Catholic priest to administer last rites. Now we more often write "a DNR."

DYING IN OLD AGE

Many people feel that large amounts of resources are spent on people as they die, and that most of Medicare funds are wasted on people who die soon. The correct figure is that 29 percent of Medicare funds go to people who die in that calendar year (Lubitz 1984). A similar number of people spend the same amount of money but do not die in that year. It is very difficult to sort out in advance which persons whose care costs a great deal will survive and which ones will not. Nevertheless, in SUPPORT, the patients whose odds of survival were very poor were already dying quickly and without life-sustaining treatments (Teno 1994). Much more variation in treatments occurs in the care of persons with more mid-range prognoses.

In sum, what can any of us expect if we die when we are old? Mostly, the answer has not been described. However, some of what we do know we try not to acknowledge. If present patterns prevail (Kemper 1991), one in every two women who live through mid-life will spend substantial time in a nursing home before they die. Among men, the rate will be about one in three, because men marry younger women and because wives and daughters take care of them. Being in a nursing home is a highly predictable event, more common than any "medical condition" except death itself. Yet consider how little time we spend worrying about the quality of nursing home care.

How does society settle on what will be spent on care in a nursing home? For that matter, how do we decide what will be spent on hospital care? Until recently, hospital payments were set at whatever the market would bear. But nursing home rates are set by scandal. Nursing home reimbursements are established by the Medicaid rate, which is set by the states each year. Every year, that rate fails to grow as much as inflation or as the need for services requires. After seven, eight, or perhaps ten years—depending on the inflation rate and how much cross-subsidization comes from private payments—the usual nursing home caring for the usual patient can no longer take care of some patients well enough to avoid scandal. Thereupon some nursing home in some big state is found to be an abyss of near abuse, others are found to be as bad, administrators and state officials lose their jobs, state commissions investigate, and the rates go up—in that state and in many others. Afterward adequate care is routinely possible for a few years again. What a clever way to establish how we are going to be cared for at the end of life! Surely some reasonably thoughtful group could have figured out a way to set what it ought to cost to take care of people who can't brush their teeth. But we haven't done it. And if we don't correct this oversight, we will live to endure the effects of that failure.

AN AGENDA FOR ACTION

So what should be done now to improve the care of the dying? First, we should attend to our language: how we establish myths and metaphors, how we structure our problems. There's no term that is more vacuous and misleading than "the terminally ill." The difference between being mortal and being terminally ill is a very hard line to find. The arrogance of establishing a category of "other" that is called "terminally ill" is a way of distancing ourselves from the fact that we're all dying. We will probably die of a chronic illness and we will probably know the cause of that death for years beforehand. Unless we improve the way we take care of people, we probably will have no one who acknowledges that death is approaching, who manages it or helps us with it.

Hospice is not the answer. Consider how our society established the Medicare hospice benefit. Not only do we have no settled approach to prognostication, but we've effectively required the patient to have a cancer with a predictable terminal phase, a home, and an unpaid family caregiver. We established a substantial public benefit aimed to serve middle-class people with predictable causes of death. Try getting patients with Alzheimer's, congestive heart failure, or cirrhosis into hospice care! Or try to enroll somebody who has no home or no caregiver. A hospice program cannot be financially viable if it accepts large numbers of people who do not have homes, caregivers, or highly predictable prognoses of short survival.

A further approach to helping the dying would be to provide palliative care much more sensibly and comprehensively. I do not want to see us "stop treatment and switch to palliative care." I want palliative care all the time. If I have a broken arm, I don't want it to hurt anymore than it has to. At some point in the course of serious disease, there may be nothing to do for me other than palliative care. But palliative care is always appropriate, even in the context of those expected to live for a long time. I want to live as long as I can, as well as I can, and I want to make the trade-offs when I must, in a way that reflects my values. That is what virtually all of us want.

There is more that we can do to improve care of the dying. We need to teach what it is we already know and demand high quality performance. It is an outrage for people who are dying to have the levels of pain that are commonly reported. We know how to eliminate pain. It is scandalous that there are still large numbers of physicians who think there's a ceiling effect on morphine. I had a patient who required two hundred milligrams of intravenously administered dilaudid per hour so he could talk with his family and be comfortable. Most oncologists have never seen such a patient. We can teach good pain relief and can make it a part of our quality assurance as well as our board and licensure exams. We do know that we can control pain. I can promise patients that they need not ever feel pain. I can't promise them that I can get rid of their hiccups, and I can't promise them that I can deal with their nausea effectively, but I can always relieve their pain. If nothing else, I can put them under anesthesia. Using what we already know to help the dying must become a priority.

We also need to reform the health care system in fundamental ways. Why is it so hard to take care of these dying patients? It's not that we don't know how; it's that we can make money and sustain our system by keeping people in the hospital, by treating them with many interventions, and by encouraging discontinuity of care. Dying patients encounter a system dominated by concerns adverse to their interests. It is easier to get open-heart surgery than Meals on Wheels. It is easier to get antibiotics than eyeglasses, and it is certainly easier to get emergency care than to get sustaining and supportive care. In this setting, getting reasonable care for a dying person often requires a struggle and usually strong advocacy by caregivers.

Some advocate active euthanasia and physician assistance in suicide as part of a solution. It would be so easy to encourage dying persons to be dead rather than to find them services. If it were easy to get good care, whether one should be able to choose to be killed would be troubling and important. But it is not easy to get good care. In fact, it is so difficult and so unlikely that people might well seek death just because doing otherwise is so burdensome. We need not tolerate this situation. We can do better.

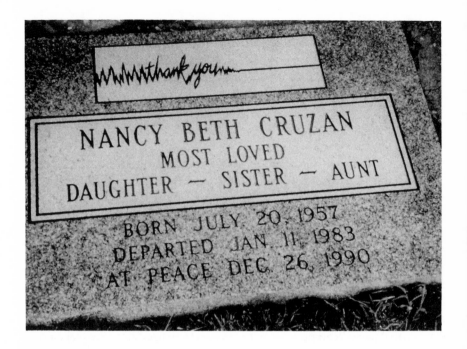

IN CLOSING

The inscription on Nancy Cruzan's tombstone reads, "Born July 20, 1957; departed January 11, 1983; at peace, December 26, 1990." Over her family's objections, Nancy Cruzan was kept alive for years while her case went through all the courts, including the Supreme Court.

The story "The Death of the Hired Man," by Robert Frost (1992), offers a contrast. The hired man, Silas, has come home to where he worked, not to his family. The farm wife has found him by the barn, huddled in a heap, and has taken him in by the fire. She meets her husband at the door and tries to explain what's happening.

> "He never did a thing so very bad.
> He don't know why he isn't quite as good
> As anyone. He won't be made ashamed
> To please his brother, worthless though he is."
>
> "I can't think Si ever hurt anyone."
> "No, but he hurt my heart the way he lay
> And rolled his old head on that sharp-edged chairback.
> He wouldn't let me put him on the lounge.

You must go in and see what you can do.
I made the bed up for him there tonight.
You'll be surprised at him—how much he's broken.
His working days are done. I'm sure of it."

"I'd not be in a hurry to say that."

"I haven't been. Go look, see for yourself.
But Warren, please remember how it is:
He's come to help you ditch the meadow.
He has a plan. You mustn't laugh at him.
He may not speak of it, and then he may.
I'll sit and see if that small sailing cloud
Will hit or miss the moon."

It hit the moon.
Then there were three there, making a dim row,
The moon, the little silver cloud, and she.
Warren returned—too soon, it seemed to her,
Slipped to her side, caught up her hand and waited.

"Warren," she questioned.
"Dead," was all he answered.

No 911, no doctor. Just an appropriate dying. A worthy goal.

References

Desbiens, N., R. E. Phillips, A. W. Wu, et al. 1994. Pain and its correlates in hospitalized patients over age 80. *Journal of General Internal Medicine* 9 (April suppl. 2): 41.
Dickinson, E. *Collected poems.* 1991. Philadelphia: Courage Books.
Frost, R. *Selected poems.* 1992. Avenel, N.J.: Gramercy Books.
Kemper, P., and C. M. Murtaugh. 1991. Lifetime use of nursing home care. *New England Journal of Medicine* 324(9): 595–600.
Knaus, W., F. Harrell, J. Lynn, et al. 1995. The SUPPORT prognostic model: Objective estimates of survival for seriously ill hospitalized adults. *Annals of Internal Medicine* 122(3): 191–203.
Lubitz, J. D., and G. F. Riley. 1993. Trends in Medicare payments in the last year of life. *New England Journal of Medicine* 328(15): 1092–96.
Lynn, J. 1993. Travels in the valley of the shadow. In *Empathy and the practice of medicine.* New Haven, Conn.: Yale University Press.

Lynn, J., J. Teno, N. Wenger, et al. 1992. "Do not resuscitate orders" in seriously ill patients: Expressed preferences or last rites? *Clinical Research* 40(2): 347a.

Lynn, J., J. M. Teno, M. T. Claessens, et al., for the SUPPORT investigators. n.d. How we die: Obstructive lung disease and lung cancer. In preparation.

Osler, W. 1904. A study of dying. Typewritten manuscript. Montreal: Bibliotheca Osleriana #7644.

Phillips, R. S., J. M. Teno, N. Wenger, et al. 1994. Elderly hospitalized patients' preferences to discuss CPR with their physicians. *Journal of General Internal Medicine* 9 (April suppl.): 41.

Pritchard, R., J. Teno, E. Fisher, et al., for the SUPPORT investigators. 1994. Regional variation in the place of death. *Journal of General Internal Medicine* 9: 146a.

SUPPORT. SUPPORT: Study to understand prognoses and preferences for outcomes and risks of treatments, study design. 1990. *Journal of Clinical Epidemiology* (suppl.): 43.

The SUPPORT Investigators. 1995. A controlled trial to improve outcomes for seriously ill hospitalized adults: The Study to Understand Prognoses and Preferences for Outcomes and Risks of Treatments (SUPPORT). *Journal of the American Medical Association,* November 22.

Teno, J. M., J. Lynn, R. S. Phillips, et al. 1994. Do formal advance directives affect resuscitation decisions and the use of resources for seriously ill patients? *Journal of Clinical Ethics* 5(1): 23–30.

Teno, J. M., D. Murphy, J. Lynn, et al. 1994. Prognosis-based futility guidelines: Does anyone win? *Journal of the American Geriatric Society* 42: 1202–7.

Wu, A. W., A. M. Damiano, J. Lynn, et al. 1995. Predicting future functional states for seriously ill hospitalized adults: The SUPPORT model. *Annals of Internal Medicine* 122: 342–50.

Chapter 11

Living in the Maelstrom

Alvin Novick

As many are well aware, gay liberation was born on June 27, 1969, in response to one of many harsh police raids on a gay social club in New York's Greenwich Village. For the first time the men who were harassed, and their friends and neighbors, fought back against irrational oppression. In consequence, we witnessed during the 1970s and into the early 1980s an exuberant liberation of spirit and a joy of living. For many gay men it was the first time in their lives that they dared exit from a deep, dark closet of camouflage, exclusion, and disrespect. In earlier years, there had not been, in any real sense, a gay community of shared interests except perhaps in a few unusual cities such as San Francisco. Not surprisingly, liberation coalesced around freedom of sexual expression—freedom to love, to relate, to express passion, and to revel in joyous self-recognition, pride, and defiance. Gay men discovered that they could express themselves openly and could develop their own styles of sexual fulfillment. They increasingly created safe spaces in which to do so.

As with most revolutions, and this was truly a revolution, excesses occurred. In this case, the revolutionaries focused on free sexuality in defiance of harsh heterosexual disdain. By the late 1970s a gay community structure, fueled by sexual liberation, began to develop around civil rights, pride, community-based service, sports, the arts, and even the professions. At that very time, however, HIV secretly and surreptitiously reached our shores, though its ravages were not recognized until 1981. What a catastrophic confluence of events—one so joyous, the other so deadly.

By the late 1970s I was already in late middle age. I had spent my adolescence, young adulthood, and middle age in a very constraining, oppressive world. A gay underground was sometimes accessible but always under nasty, almost unthinkably cruel circumstances. We of these earlier generations slowly came out, came to feel some elements of pride, came to love ourselves and to be capable of loving other men, but we were always under clouds of disrespect. As liberation reached its height, I was already in my mid-fifties—well beyond what one might envision as a sexually active or easily marketable age. Largely through my life partner, Bill, who was twenty years younger than I and much more gay-aware, I came to witness the joyousness of liberation and of sexual liberation and the incredibly fulfilling possibility of being a professor, a physician, and an openly gay and proud man all at the same time.

Almost all of the men I came to know and came to honor and share my existence with were Bill's age. Most of the men of my age were retiring and retired or could not shed their camouflage. In consequence, on vacations, in social life, and in my growing gay professional life I came to meet and be surrounded by vibrant, beautiful, wonderful men in their thirties or forties. And in 1982, when I started a new career as a gay and as an AIDS advocate and activist, I rapidly met a substantial cross section of similarly evolving colleagues—including health care providers, lawyers, writers, creative artists, and activists of every class and skill—who were almost all in their thirties or forties. Away from Yale, away from my traditional roles, these were the men with whom I played, worked, intrigued, and created.

They are almost all dead or dying.

A very high proportion of urban gay men who were out and proud in the 1970s were infected with HIV before its existence was known. The very same men made up the core of those who did, and are doing, almost all of the AIDS and gay advocacy in America. The same men shaped the community's response, developed services, spoke out, led protests, cared for the ill, shaped much of national public policy, articulated prevention messages, and fought for all of their fellow assailed communities—the intravenous drug users, inner-city people of color, sex workers, blood transfusion recipients, men with hemophilia, and babies.

I became part of an international network of daring, wondrous heroes and a parallel network of their spouses and friends. These defiant and committed men are largely going or gone—lost heroes by tens of thousands.

In San Francisco currently about 70 percent of "older" gay men—those who were in their thirties and forties fifteen years ago—are HIV infected. Many more have succumbed. Of younger gay men, 30 to 50 percent are also infected, dying, or dead. I've come to know and treasure many of them as well. I see them and remember them with love, respect, honor, and despair.

My lengthy introduction is not intended to be self-indulgent. I have to convey the concept—all but impossible for "others" to feel, either emotionally or cerebrally—what this maelstrom of loss means.

This epidemic is now at least eighteen to twenty years old. There is no sign of its abating. The threat of illness and death embeds every gay urban youth and young adult, as well as those middle-aged men who remain well. AIDS, we now know, is not a short-term crisis. It will surely span the lifetime of those who are now young adults. The average life expectancy for gay youths in San Francisco has recently been projected to be only forty-five years.

The previously secret HIV epidemic became an immediate crisis by 1982–85. Now it is far beyond an acute crisis; it is a permeating fact of life and of death. Gay men have died in their prime, and they will continue to do so for one or two generations to come. And those who still survive and those who will survive envision a black and tenuous future, a devalued life span, a devalued life. Communities of uninfected men are hopeless, forlorn, isolated, assailed by loss and grief, anxious, uncertain, depressed, and often consumed with guilt and survivor guilt. They often live their lives as if they are dying. And we damage them more—not simply because we fail to bolster their pride, enhance their self-image, value them, or join hands with them in their grief and agitation. No. Our failure is more paradoxical than that: we preach simple, deeply demanding, and often hostile and demeaning messages. Not infrequently these messages are meant in good faith, but they are often truly devilish. And they are usually homophobic and debasing of gay love, affection, sexuality, and spirituality. Our messages infringe on the very lives that men already perceive to be futile but that often are all the more futile because we drain or deplete them of their richness.

Few of us have become accustomed to the deaths of young men or women. Few of us can conjecture about the meaning of lost futures—not just the lost futures of those who are dead or dying (as would be the case for those who die in combat), but also the lost futures of those who are well: those who live in a disappearing community embedded in an unsupportive, hostile, or indifferent society.

I have come to know all these things. I hear these pains. I sorrow for gay youth who mourn for lives they will not fill. And I fight to give these youngsters back their futures. I cannot produce the cure or the vaccine. I can, however, love and honor them. I can share my pride with them. And I can express hope and try to help them feel valued and valuable enough to invest in life—even in a dark life. Without them, all our lives will be darker.

I have known many men who long to become infected so that they can envision and plan a known future—a future of sharing and support. I see envy, guilt, and resignation. Maybe you do, too. It's time to restore and share those futures. It's time for us to be creative and decent—all of us. We must not foster their hope to regain their lives by becoming infected with a fatal virus—to regain life by committing to death!

In 1982, at the first public forum on AIDS that I attended, a devoted HIV physician closed by reading off a list of the first names of those he had already lost—perhaps twenty-five in all. The effect was riveting. I can no longer do that. The list is too long, too laden with grief.

On World AIDS Day this past December, I attended a service in memory of those from New Haven that we have lost to the epidemic. Their names were read off. It took about an hour. How moving it was to hear the names of so many people I had come to know and treasure, with whom I had shared personal, professional, and advocacy adventures. How devastating; how cathartic; how painful. And these were largely my other network of brothers and sisters—injection drug users, people of color, heterosexuals, and babies.

My address book is now empty. When I'm troubled I have almost no one to call who would understand, and almost all of those few who are alive are ill or are caring for a dying lover or friend. I dare not burden them with my sorrow.

I've been focusing our attention on the troubled living, the well, and the dead and dying. Let us take another look at those who are HIV infected and know or believe themselves to be so. These men and women would seem to have had their worst fears come true. That surely is true of many but not of all. For some the diagnosis comes in some ways as a relief of tension, a clarification of futility, or a march down fate's pathway. For others, whatever their initial devastation and confusion may be, their known and shared destiny comes to shape their lives into defiance (sometimes combined with denial) and inspires them to engage in fierce advocacy or in service delivery. They often exceed all reasonable expectations. Were we speaking in spiritual terms, I would easily classify many of the men and women I have known as saintly in their altruistic service. Some, it seems to me, are Christ-like. Many are militantly independent and channel everything they've got to serve out their shortened life with glory and productivity. Many others seem to wish to be quiet role models of almost any wonderful behavior: of kindness, leadership, activism, brilliance, incendiary poetry or prose, creativity in dance or theater. All of these things and more. Why are people so brave in the face of horrible deaths and demeaning deterioration? I leave it to others to develop full scholarly explanations, but let me offer a few lay insights of my own. For one, I believe it may be fulfilling, in a sense, for severely oppressed and disdained people to feel punished. Gay men are part of the same homophobic society that so scorns them. Perhaps there's an ultimate liberation that flows from this master stroke of cruelty that society has helped focus on them.

Second, I perceive that many of us relish a chance to be better, braver, more sensitive, and more tasteful than heterosexuals—to show off how good we are. Note the possibilities of parallel interpretations of much of Jewish behavior under oppression. HIV disease does offer a great variety of showcases for "goodness" that need not be fully overtly occupied. That is, one can rise to the occasion of illness and death publicly (or privately) without necessarily being ill publicly.

Third, many men and women actually discover a power in being fatally ill that enables them to do wonderful things. They may feel, or even actually be empowered by their new focus and by an enlightened daring that comes from knowing their life spans will be brief.

How many outsiders can have taken time to perceive that not only are there many openly infected heroic advocates, activists, and creators of key services, but that most of the other altruists of the HIV setting are infected as well? Those who are ill are doing the work, and perhaps, if we're lucky in some sense, that's who *will* be doing the work. Have we ever really seen that phenomenon before?

In the final days or weeks of life (and for some the final months) the setting shifts. Even gay or AIDS activists—or saints—have to die. I've witnessed more than my share of these deaths. The most troubled have been for those men who have lost their self-selected family. Many of those in the worst trouble have had to return to their birth families because they could no longer support independent lives. The problem is not always cruel judgment. More often, I believe, no one in their birth family knows who they are and where they've been. These men then die alone.

We have come to know death, as well as bravery, resilience, and glorious defiance. We've seen incredible altruism. But wondrous men and women are still being struck down and will continue to be for one or two more generations at least. Many of us can no longer feel enough anger, grief, love, and hope. Every one of us and every one of them needs these things, but most of all we need, increasingly, safe space, regard, and respect. We need to feel treasured. We still die spurned.

What are we to do?

The virus creates new and horrible ways for men and women to die, and many of our most promising new drugs actually raise the horror level. We, the gay men who survive, are inventing new ways to be supportive and encompassing. We are even inventing new ways of easing death. Yet few others recognize our efforts or ask us to teach them how they too can contribute.

What are you to do?

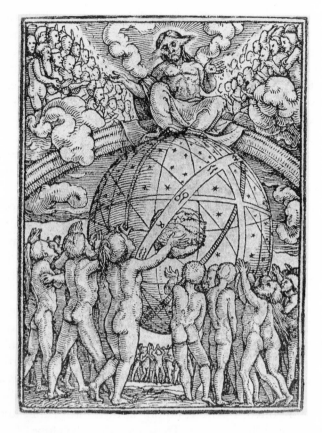

Hans Holbein the Younger, *The Last Judgment,* woodcut. Rosenwald Collection © 1995 Board of Trustees, National Gallery of Art, Washington, D.C.

Part 2 Framing Death: Cultural and Religious Responses

Lee Palmer Wandel

The image that prefaces this section belongs to the visual tradition of the Dance of Death, which exploded in popularity in the late Middle Ages and Renaissance in Europe. Before turning to the chapters in this part, I invite you to pause over that image and, by extension, the others in this volume and on its cover. This particular image is a woodcut from the series the German Renaissance artist Hans Holbein the Younger designed for a volume of *The Dance of Death*, which—because of his beautiful and wry illustrations—would become the most popular version of all time. It is an image of the Last Judgment. It represents concepts for which we have no biological data: the judgment of souls, salvation, eternity, life after death. Its content is entirely "fictive"—in other words, by the empirical standards of science, it is the product not of research, but of imagination, culture, belief.

And yet the moment that the Holbein woodcut sought to represent—souls of the dead standing before Christ the Judge in the last moment of human time—had a certain reality not only for sixteenth-century readers of *The Dance of Death*, but for Christians throughout time and across the globe. The notion of a final judgment of each human life was developed perhaps most fully in Christian theology and art, where literature, sculpture, and paintings described in words and images the moment when divinity sits in judgment over each human life, rewarding and punishing in some sort of "life" after death, heaven or hell, to which each would be assigned for eternity. But many religious and cultural traditions hold a notion of final and perfect judgment in which death is the opening, the portal, not the end. They conceive of death, in other words, as some sort of transition from one kind of "life" to another. As we shall see, for early American Puritans, in Judaism, Catholicism, and Islam, "life" does not end with the cessation of breath or neurological function; for these religions, and in late medieval Chinese popular belief, death is bound up with justice; in Chinese popular beliefs and in Christianity, true justice is often realized only after death; in Islam, the cities of the dead jostle cities of the living; and for Christianity, Islam, and Hinduism, "souls" confound any clear division between life and death.

This section thus takes up not the fact of death, but its meaning within the larger reference of human life—not the biology of death, but cultural and religious meditations on its place in our understanding of ourselves as human. Much more than birth, marriage, or other events in the passage of a life, death has been the focus of religious and cultural reflection. Across centuries, languages, and continents, religions as diverse as Hinduism and Catholicism and cultures as different as those found in seventeenth-century New England and medieval China have all provided frames of meaning for death—ways of thinking of it and of placing it in a larger world view. In this section, an anthropologist, historians, theologians, and pastors describe some of those other ways of conceiving of death—as portal, as negotiated with God, as essential to human life, as a moment in which one's future in an afterlife is manifested.

The first chapter in this part, by the demographic historian Arthur Imhof, returns us to the late medieval *ars moriendi,* the art of dying, which was practiced by Christians throughout the Continent. It offered stages for the dying and those attending, ways to move from the world of the living through a peaceful death in the hope of reaching purgatory or heaven—in other words, ways to find a "good death." Imhof argues passionately for the importance of returning to these older ways of framing death in order to find, in this age of aggressive medicine and secular conceptions of life, a "good death."

The remaining chapters all courageously take up an impossible enterprise. In the brief space allotted to each author, it would not have been possible to render in its fullness any of the cultures' or religions' conceptions of the meaning of death. None of the essays, therefore, is exhaustive of the religion or culture it discusses. Instead a number of the scholars chose to offer vignettes, windows into other ways of thinking about death. Valerie Hansen chooses a single life, the late medieval Chinese man Liu Yuan Balang who brought back knowledge and evidence of the world of the spirits, while John Demos sketches the death scenes of two very different early American women, Mrs. Forbush and Sarah Lippet, each surrounded by family and attended by her pastor, each the star of this elemental scene. Both carry us eloquently into very different worlds of meaning. Some offer impressions drawn from a lifetime of research: Sylvia Vatuk delineates the touchstones of Hindu thinking on death, while Harald Wagner summarizes the central tenets of Catholicism on the topics of death and the afterlife. Ira Lapidus provides a rich portrait of Islamic understandings of death, mourning, funerals, and the place of the dead in the lives of the living. James Ponet provides Talmudic meditations on death in the Jewish tradition. Peter Hawkins offers an eloquent meditation on the AIDS Memorial Quilt and the importance not only of acts of commemoration and memorialization, but also of private acts of memory. His is at once a deeply humane acknowledgment of the suffering of those who must witness and an encouragement to give grief itself aesthetic form—to "name" the person one has lost to death.

William McCullough, surgeon and former Presbyterian minister, and Frederick Streets, the Yale University chaplain, seek to bridge in different ways the distance that has grown between medicine and religion. McCullough reflects on the interfaces between and the tensions dividing medicine and theology, suggesting avenues of communication between these two different professions with their attendant sets of attitudes. Streets invites doctors to attend the funerals of their patients, not only to acknowledge and respect the beliefs and religious commitments of their patients, but also to participate in the different traditions' forms of grieving as a way of reinforcing their connection with the family and of recognizing and articulating their own grief at the loss of a patient.

For doctors, these essays may be among the most important. Each offers a beautifully colored sketch of a distinctive, perhaps unfamiliar, context of meaning for death. In doing so, these essays set forth an array of ways of "framing" death, for returning it to its context of human life, for giving the fact of death meaning within the far larger framework of human creativity, activity, life. They offer paths to move from a view of death as the "failure" of care or cure to a more integrative understanding of death as an essential, and for some definitive, part of the whole of human existence—a fulcrum of meaning. In so doing, perhaps these essays will help us to recover that sense, expressed by Sir James Barrie in *Peter Pan,* that "to die will be a great adventure."[1]

Note

1. Quoted on the Order of Service for the funeral of Nancy Bateson Nisbet Rash, Thursday, March 16, 1995.

Chapter 12

An *Ars Moriendi* for Our Time:
To Live a Fulfilled Life; to Die a Peaceful Death

Arthur E. Imhof

Of all living beings, we humans are the only ones who know that we must die, and who can view our end with calm. For most of us, however, that is a difficult position for two main reasons. First, we have lost our immortality: only a very few still have an unqualified belief in the resurrection of the dead and in eternal life. Second, our demise in this world is made even more problematic because the number of our descendants has so dramatically shrunk and many of us do not have any children at all. How then can we live on, at least for a time, in their memories?

LIFE AND DEATH IN OUR TIME

In general, we are very proud of the fact that our average life expectancy has doubled or even tripled within a few generations. If something happens to one of us prematurely, he or she can usually be promptly repaired. We believe it is our right to feel nearly immortal during our "best years." A slew of prevention campaigns insinuate that we may indeed soon attain immortality: with a little more jogging, no more smoking, rigorous stair climbing, consumption of low-fat milk, and regular "check-ups," it might be possible to put death off altogether. Once upon a time illnesses carried meaning with them. They were taken as a benign hint from God to stop our sinful ways in time. What sense, if any, do health problems make nowadays? They certainly no longer have their old meaning. And yet they often provide the only chance in our hectic lives to turn inward and reflect. Are we afraid we will not find anything in there, within ourselves?

Paradoxically, death's permanent presence in the media contributes to its sterility. The media show deaths, but only those that occur under unusual circumstances, which we find easy to discount as irrelevant to our own lives. Few of us will die a newsworthy death in a plane crash, during an earthquake, under a collapsed skyscraper or a mine, or during a terrorist attack. But even if our own deaths in all likelihood will be banal, we should not ignore death or consider it insignificant. Who among us would want to trade a quiet death for one of those millions of horrible deaths inflicted by human hands during two world wars, in concentration and prison camps, in bombings and firestorms? Today, at least most of us die a natural death.

Death in our time has become a more modest presence, leaving most of us in peace for decades, even if it ultimately prevails. Yet even under these totally new conditions, we find it hard to achieve a balance in our lives, for living means to accept the tension of becoming, being, and decaying that is in us from the start. Balance means not only to accept and endure this tension but to give it meaning and shape. Moreover, for laymen and health professionals alike it means to accept a natural death at the right moment, and not to prevent it—which, technically, has become possible to do temporarily. The old dream of a fulfilled and completed life goes back in our culture to the philosophers of antiquity. That this dream is now suddenly becoming true for more and more people is something totally new. No wonder that many still have problems with it.

If, as they say, the one life we have is our finest possession, and it used to last thirty or forty years, what shall we do with the additional thirty or forty years we now have? Not everyone seems to know. Certainly there is suicide at all stages of life. But suicide grows more common in people over seventy, as suicide researchers and gerontologists confirm. Gained years are not necessarily fulfilled years. We have to fill them with meaning. If people spend their lives interested only in physical activity but not in spiritual-cultural matters, they should not be surprised to find themselves confronting a great spiritual emptiness when their physical powers wane in old age and they do not know how to fill the extra days, months, and years. But this need not be so: the situation could be prevented with a lifelong cultivation of spiritual and artistic interests.

Our dilemma is this: the doubling, even tripling of our life expectancy is only one side of the coin. The other side is that along with the increase of our earthly life expectancy there has been a totally different, countervailing development. The result is that over the last generations our lives have by no means become longer, but have instead—because of the loss of faith in the Beyond—become *infinitely* shorter. Doesn't the doubling of our earthly years mean little in relation to the loss of faith in an eternity?

Against this background we need not be astonished that most of us go through life in reverse, as it were, with our backs turned on old age and dying. We worship youth because it is at the furthest remove from the final exit. One can understand why the body as the only guarantee of our remaining earthly life is valued so highly once an afterlife has been rationalized away. When our body is no more, we are no more. Therefore we watch our bodies incessantly, cultivate and pamper them, do bodybuilding and everything else to ensure their smooth functioning.

Even if most of us live the full extent of our natural lifespans, we remain mortal, and that is not a *medical* problem. It is not a problem at all, but a part of our humanity. Who are we, among all living beings, to alone claim immortality? If medical science attempted to prevent death, that would be inhuman. The problem is that many of us think that medical science should continue to be in charge even when nothing more can be done and nothing more should be done. Death is *not* a medical teaching subject, and dying right is not part of medical studies. Here a vacuum exists with both professionals and lay people, because instruction in dying right is not required for anybody, in whatever discipline. We are all alone in that regard. Although all of us will die, hardly anyone is prepared, or is preparing, to die right. It used to be quite different.

OUR ANCESTORS LEARNED HOW TO DIE

Let us look back to the second half of the fifteenth century. By then, printmaking techniques permitted the relatively inexpensive production of woodcuts in large editions that could be distributed cheaply. It had long been the task of priests to help the dying through their last hours. The problem, however, was that during the frequent epidemics many people died at the same time, and there were not enough priests to assist everyone. The priests also knew from experience, just like the "loved ones" of the sick, that contagious diseases were extremely dangerous. Whoever could flee did so, and the farther the better. In short, nobody could be certain of not having to die alone.

What did our forebears do? They *learned* to die, everyone for him- or herself, even when they were still young. Even if they could not read, they could look at woodcuts. In the view of that time, a soul's fate was often decided during the last hour on earth. It was thought that the devil's forces would try everything to get hold of the soul about to depart. People of those times could imagine what these final temptations would be: tempting of the faith, tempting into despair, and tempting into impatience, pride and arrogance, and earthly materialism. Whoever succumbed to one of these hellish temptations in that last hour was certain to forfeit the heavenly splendors and suffer in eternal hell.

A typical small educational brochure consisted of eleven woodcuts. In each picture the dying person was shown in bed, an Everyman of about forty, with whom all could identify. Five woodcuts illustrated the five great temptations already mentioned. Terrible devils' faces bear down on the *moribundus* from all sides. They show him his register of sins and let all his life's misdeeds parade by. As perjuror, adulterer, miser, drunkard, glutton, thief, and murderer, he would stand no chance of God's mercy. The wood-cuts would appeal also to his vanity, would flatter him, remind him of his life's accomplishments, the honors, heroic deeds, and fame. They would mention all his possessions, to distract him from concentrating on dying in a way that would please God.

The corresponding images on another five woodcuts, however, showed the heavenly forces hurrying to his side: angels, saints, and the Trinity. They supported the dying person in his struggle for the soul. Five times he would resist with their help. Then he died. The eleventh woodcut would show the happy end: an angel ready to receive the expired soul in the shape of a small naked child and lead it into God's heavenly splendor.

Dying, the *right* way of dying, could be learned. If one had absorbed this *ars bene moriendi*, this "art of dying right" at a young age, one no longer had to fear dying, not even dying alone. One knew what the last hour would hold in store, and one only had to copy Everyman on the woodcuts to be assured eternal bliss.

As a historian, I am always tempted to look at how our forebears dealt with problems like ours today. Just as in the past, nobody can be sure that he or she will not have to spend the last hour without spiritual help and die alone. But who teaches *us* how to die?

AN *ARS MORIENDI* FOR OUR TIME

No one is so naive as to suggest republishing the old *Ars Moriendi* and distributing it in large numbers to people to help them relearn the "art of dying right." But if we agree that even in our time once again we need an *ars moriendi*—and I believe we do—there are some good lessons to be learned from the old.

First, an *ars moriendi* should be rooted in its time. Half a millennium ago it was based, as a matter of course, in the Christian world view and its belief in a Beyond, in resurrection and eternal life. It prepared one for the struggle for the soul in the last hour and guaranteed a successful outcome to those who followed its precepts. For most of us today, life consists only of its earthly part. The process of dying rings in the final chapter.

Second, a decisive factor in the success of the earlier *ars moriendi* was its concentration on the essential. Eleven expressive, understandable wood-cuts sufficed to make the point. A contemporary *ars moriendi* must also be concise and poignant, as well as generally accessible. It must speak to *everyone* today, just like long ago, for once again nobody can be sure of not dying alone.

Third, the "art of dying alone" addressed everyone, even in their early years, for nobody could be certain about not having to die alone the very next day. Thus, the *ars moriendi* was also an *ars vivendi*, an "art of living right." Living such a fulfilled earthly life means that at its natural end we are willing to let go even without the prospect of any continuation.

To begin this learning process only with the loss of health and the prospect of death is usually much too late. Just like five hundred years ago, the practice has to begin in youth. Thus, this new *ars moriendi* is not a manual for intensive care units, hospice, or the bedroom at home. The motto of this *ars* is to "live fulfilled," to do so all of one's life and as a result "to die in peace." The last weeks, days, or hours may turn out to be whatever and wherever, no matter what illness leads to my end or whether I die without help in a hospital, in a nursing home, or at home. I have lived my life and did not just grow older. Fulfilled by life, and not just tired of it, I can give it up.

Being open-minded about our situation today makes it easier to find solutions. To be open-minded means to not only take note of the following facts, but also draw conclusions from them. For example, we can read that the average life expectancy in Germany was 37.2 years in 1855, whereas it was 74.6 years in 1985, an exact doubling. Further, not only do we have twice as many years, we also have twice as many good years. Our nutrition is more assured and better than ever before. Infectious diseases are largely under control. We work half as long as our ancestors and generally under better conditions. Economically, with some exceptions, we can afford many more things. Information of all kinds—obtained through numerous television and radio channels, an overabundance of print media, museums, libraries, concert halls, and universities all over the world—is available to all of us as never before.

Are all these advantages worth nothing to us? Dozens of generations before us have striven for a long life. We have it. We are living a dream come true for humankind. And yet we are insatiable—we want more years, better years, and, if possible, all of eternity as well.

To be sure, the current control over "plague, hunger, and war" and the resulting increase in life span to an age never before achieved are not guaranteed forever. New plagues threaten us, such as AIDS or wars in different parts of the world. How long this unusual state will last depends in large measure on our vigilance and on our willingness to contribute. The historian knows plenty of examples of stagnating, even regressive life ex-pectancy. I don't want to paint images of horror; for some, such images qualify the change from an insecure to a secure lifetime and bring about a free-floating anxiety that is hard to conquer. It is a mistake to let fear paralyze you.

The fact is that of today's 80 million or so Germans, more than half were born after 1950. Thus for the first time a large stratum of German society has not experienced the immediate threats of "plague, hunger, and war" that reigned for millennia. For the first time the *majority* of the German population has been given the astounding opportunity of living and shaping their lives in terms of a quasi-calculable end. This offers an amazing chance to realize a life plan. For the first time we can weigh and coordinate the strengths and weaknesses of each phase of our lives. It no longer makes sense to live just from one day to the next. Given the already mentioned weakening of our physical abilities, it is important to cultivate from early youth not only physical but also intellectual and cultural interests, both in oneself and in others, so that one finds pleasure in each phase of life and makes the last years worth living.

Even for those who still die early, as victims of accidents or incurable diseases, the realization of a life plan makes sense, I think, even if it is cut short. Everything happened for them, too, at the right time. Dying young or old, nobody should berate him- or herself on the deathbed for having missed something. There should be no last-minute, panicky attempt to catch up on what cannot be recouped. The goal should be "to live fulfilled—to die serenely," at whatever age.

CONCLUSION

Have we been assuming that the change from an uncertain to a certain life expectancy will bring with it an earthly paradise? Only naive people ignore the two sides of a coin.

Let's weigh the facts. Developments since World War II have brought us much that is positive, particularly the shift from an uncertain to a certain life span. We have twice as many years, we have twice as many good years, we can afford more things than ever, and we have more access to the world than ever before. But the same development has brought us gravely negative changes: the widespread loss of faith in eternity, the possibility of prolonged illness, and the decay of our communal structures, to name just a few.

I doubt that anyone would like to rescind these negative developments by returning to the bad old days of "plague, hunger, and war." We are free to do so. The old infectious diseases have not disappeared from the face of the earth. Hunger and war still exist. Everybody is free to travel without prophylaxis into malaria-infested areas, to go without preserved foodstuffs into the African or Asian hunger zones, or to visit theaters of war. He or she would find the desired premature death and would never have to think about life plans or a new *ars moriendi*.

Most of us, however, embrace the long life that has finally become possible, and we must accept its concomitant negatives. Let us make the best of the long life we have wished so hard for and that we are now privileged to have. Let us transform every one of the years gained into fulfilled ones, taking advantage of our immense technical, economic, and cultural resources, and then let us die a natural death.

As I wrote at the beginning of this chapter, to be human is to accept and meaningfully endure the tension within us from the beginning—the tension between becoming and being, between being and perishing. Is that so hard to comprehend? Concise and brief, like the old *ars moriendi,* this is an essential truth for all of us.

Note

More on the topic of this contribution can be found in the author's interactive CD-ROM *Ars moriendi,* (Stuttgart: Wissenschaftliche Verlagsgesellschaft, 1995).

Chapter 13

The Art of Dying in Hindu India

Sylvia Vatuk

I originally became interested in the question of Hindu approaches to dying while doing anthropological research on the cultural and social dimensions of aging in northern India. Although biological aging is a human universal, how people think about old age, the manner in which they cope with physical decline and social losses in later life, and the positions they occupy in relation to family and society vary a great deal from one culture to another. There is also great cultural diversity in the way people deal with death and dying—a fact that provides the central theme of this book.

My own research was carried out in the 1970s in a major Indian city, among a population with very recent rural origins. Among these people I found attitudes toward aging and death that seemed much more positive than our own. There was a greater degree of acceptance of the inevitability of mortality, and more attention was given to preparing actively for the end of life. While the material circumstances of their lives were far less comfortable than our own, these people seemed better equipped, both cognitively and emotionally, to face the inevitability of aging, dying, and death. It would be foolish to idealize or romanticize the situation of older people in India. It would be misleading to suggest that for them the later years of life are free from stress or that their deaths are free from fear, suffering, and pain. Indians and Westerners alike are all too prone to accept the familiar stereotype of the "spiritual" Hindu who consistently treats his elders with the loving care, honor, and respect that his culture and religion prescribe. The reality, of course, is far more complex than this ideal. Nevertheless, there are real differences between Indian and American ways of aging and death. For Hindus these are grounded in certain key cultural conceptions about the nature of the world, human life, and the social order.[1]

A central cosmological concept is that of *samsara*—"transmigration" or "reincarnation." All sentient beings are believed to belong to a continuum of life forms, from the most lowly insect to the highest living form, the human being. Birth, life, and death are part of a never-ending cyclical process. While the material body is mortal, the individual "soul" (*atman*) is eternal—at death it separates from the body and is reborn, after a period of time, in the body of another living being.

The ultimate goal of the soul is to escape from this cycle of rebirths, to attain *moksha*—"liberation" or "release"—and become reabsorbed into the oneness of the Universal Soul. The soul's direction and rate of progress toward *moksha* depend upon how those beings in whose ephemeral bodies the soul is housed live their worldly lives. The causal principle is that of *karma*—"action." Simply put, good actions lead to the accumulation of "merit" (*punya*) and speed one's soul toward its ultimate release; bad deeds cause the accumulation of "sin" (*pap*) and retard the soul's progress toward this desired end.

The circumstances into which one is born and the kind of experiences one has in life are also understood to depend upon one's accumulated *karma*. Good *karma* from prior lives brings happiness and good fortune in this life, while the consequence of bad *karma* is misery and suffering. Likewise, one's behavior in this life has consequences, for good or ill, in lives to come. If through one's deeds one contributes toward the soul's store of *punya*, one may hope for rebirth into a higher social station in the next life; one who commits evil deeds will suffer in the next life, in the extreme case being denied human rebirth and taking the form of some lower animal.[2]

There are said to be three possible "paths" toward liberation from the cycle of rebirths: selfless action, religious devotion, and spiritual knowledge. One may choose the path or paths that best suit one's capabilities or inclinations, but all are long and arduous. Only through the most exceptional exertions can a person attain release for the soul in the course of a single lifetime. Spiritual knowledge is generally regarded as the superior path. Through it one comes to appreciate the Oneness of ultimate reality and recognizes the false or illusory nature of the phenomenal world. As long as one remains "caught in the net of *maya*" (illusion), one's soul cannot attain *moksha*. To reach this level of spiritual understanding, it is necessary to cease involvement in worldly activities, cares, and concerns, with the ultimate aim of extricating oneself completely from all interpersonal attachments.

Acceptance of the notions of *karma* and *maya* is not inconsistent with an active approach to death. On the contrary, it is imperative that an aging Hindu prepare him- or herself appropriately for departing the world. In

Madan's words, "The ultimate and critical sign of the good life may be available in the manner a person attains his death" (1988, 122). The phrase "attain death" is crucial. The Hindu is urged to actively participate in setting the proper stage for his own dying.

A good death is one in which the dying person is in full possession of his or her mental and physical faculties and is fully cognizant of what is about to be experienced. There is time to assume the proper frame of mind for what is to come and to take adequate leave of family and friends. One is not overtaken by death but "lets go of life" deliberately and willingly. In contrast, "the 'bad' death is one for which the deceased cannot be said to have prepared himself. It is said that 'he did not die his own death'" (Parry 1982, 83). In the Hindu view, in contrast to our own, the sudden, painless death of an elderly person—as from a heart attack or stroke—is not regarded as a fortunate one, for the deceased had no time to ready himself for this most crucial passage. Deaths by accident or other violent means are regarded with even greater horror, both for this reason and also because of fears that the victim's embittered spirit may return as a ghost to afflict the living.

Only a person who has lived a long and full life can be said to die a good death; thus death ought properly to come in old age, not in childhood or youth. Ideally, one's spouse, children—including at least one son—and grandchildren should be alive and present at the deathbed. Death should come at home or at one of the sacred Hindu pilgrimage sites. Banaras is especially favored, for it is said that the souls of all who die in that holy city immediately attain *moksha* (Parry 1994, 27).

A person who senses that death is approaching should inform family members, refuse further nourishment, and be lifted from the bed to a spot on the ground that has been ritually purified for the purpose. Those present should read aloud some appropriate holy text or sing devotional songs to help fix the mind of the dying person upon the Divine. Then, at a moment deliberately chosen, the dying man or woman takes a final breath. When a very old person dies in this way, leaving many surviving descendants, his or her funerary rites are observed not with outward expressions of sadness but with a colorful and celebratory procession and joyous feasting in congratulatory appreciation of a life well lived and a death well died. Such a funeral is indeed often verbally and symbolically equated with a marriage party.

Hindus share a set of notions about the "ideal human life course" that are also relevant to understanding their way of death. Various ancient didactic treatises provide highly formalized and elaborated versions of a model of life stages (*ashrama*).[3] The most common textual formulation posits four of these, a man being sequentially a Student, a Householder, a

Forest-Dweller or Hermit, and a Renouncer of the world.[4] The physically
mature, married, sexually and economically active Householder is at the
center of the social order, all others being dependent upon him for suste-
nance. Occupants of the third and fourth *ashramas* are already on the social
periphery as they turn away from mundane worldly concerns and ready
themselves to depart this life.

In the words of Manu, the most well known of the ancient lawgivers,
when a Householder "sees that he is wrinkled and grey, and [sees] the
children of his children, then he should take himself to the wilderness"
(Doniger 1991, 17). Entering the third stage of life, that of the Hermit, he
hands over household affairs to his son and heir and devotes his energies to
spiritual reflection and bodily mortification. Thus he begins to disentangle
himself—physically and emotionally—from the bonds of *maya*. Having
succeeded in this, he enters the fourth and final *ashrama*, renouncing the
world completely in preparation for death.

What is the nature of the relationship between the religious conceptions
and cultural ideals that I have outlined here and the actual circumstances,
behaviors, and emotions of real individuals trying to come to terms with
the personal experience of aging and death? A prominent Indian anthropologist answers this question for the Kashmiri Brahmans he has studied:
"Death is . . . made bearable by its being treated as an opportunity for the
individual soul to realize union with 'that' [universal soul] from which it
has . . . separated" (Madan 1988, 137). But, we may ask, does such an
abstract idea as *moksha* really enable the ordinary Hindu to face death with
equanimity—any more than the notion that the soul of a virtuous man
goes to heaven allows the average Christian to contemplate life's ending
with pleasant anticipation?

In my view, the relationship between Hindu cosmology, on the one
hand, and the emotional state of those who are old and dying, on the other,
is much more complex than Madan's statement suggests. What the religious and cultural conceptions I have outlined do provide for the Hindu
man or woman is a repertoire of meaning and explanation upon which to
draw when trying to understand and cope with major life transitions. They
provide "a map for living"—and for dying—that "defines human goals,
outlines alternatives, and lays down principles" for action and thought
(Hiebert 1981, 215). Individuals use this map selectively, in ways that suit
their particular needs at particular times. Some people are more successful
than others in deriving from it a sense of direction, comfort, and solace.
Yet, however personally inclined or capable of making practical use of it in
designing their own lives and deaths, few Hindus would disagree about the
ultimate wisdom of trying to do so.

The Indian men and women I came to know in the course of my research all took for granted that the soul is involved in an eternal cycle of rebirths. They frequently cited *karma* as the main causal principle for human misfortune, though very often it was described as operating in the short term rather than over the course of a series of rebirths.[5] Thus they suggested that unkind, selfish, or immoral deeds were often punished in a person's present life, perhaps in the form of a painful final illness and a lingering death. As one old man put it, "According to the deeds a man does, so is his death. If he does good deeds, he dies easily and doesn't have to suffer much pain. He who does bad deeds, who commits sins, gives pain to others, God gives the fruits of that right here." Not surprisingly, on the other hand, people tended to blame their own misfortune and suffering on "fate" or "predestination" (*bhagya*), thereby relieving themselves of the responsibility implied in the *karma* theory.

When explaining how they were preparing for their own deaths, these old people tended to emphasize the paths of religious devotion and spiritual knowledge, rather than the accumulation of merit through good deeds. This tendency is consistent with the textual view that the path of "selfless action" is most appropriate for those in the Householder stage, fully engaged as they are in worldly affairs. Many older men and women reported devoting considerably more time and effort to religious worship, contemplation, and self-reflection than they had in earlier years. The elderly were always heavily represented among those frequenting temples and gathering for devotional recitations and singing.

Older people rarely expressed a concern with improving their lot in the next life. More often they spoke about working toward that more distant goal of escaping the round of rebirths altogether. None, however, dared to hope that their meager efforts in the few years remaining to them would be sufficient to ensure the immediate attainment of their soul's ultimate goal.

The notion of a human life span divided into distinct periods—with certain activities, behaviors, concerns, and attitudes appropriate to each—provided these Hindus with a ready framework for thinking about life in general and about their own lives in particular. It provided a guide for how to act and even to feel as they progressed through the life cycle. They often made explicit reference to "life stages," asserting—in line with the textual formulation of these—that in old age one should withdraw from active work and allow oneself to be housed, fed, and cared for by one's sons and daughters-in-law. They agreed that at this stage of life one should rein in one's desires and follow an ascetic regimen, cultivate an attitude of indifference to food, dress simply, and eschew worldly forms of enjoyment, particularly sexual expression. In practice, most older men and women appeared to follow these prescriptions for living to a considerable degree, aided not only by the strength of their own personal inclinations but by social pressure from those around them.

The metaphors of world renunciation and escape from the net of *maya* were frequently employed when elderly men and women imparted what they considered the essence of their outlook on life. An inability to achieve peace of mind was commonly attributed to the inhibiting effect of *maya*, which makes one care excessively about household problems. As one man explained, many older people "are too much involved with their family members. Even up to the time of their death they are not able to detach themselves from the family. They keep suffering from worry over the difficulties all of them are having."

Others are more successful in cultivating detachment. Several men claimed to have already "left the world" or to have "become Renouncers," although to all appearances they were living like anyone else—residing in the bosom of the family, socializing with their peers, and taking active roles in community politics and ceremonial events. What they meant to communicate was that their *mental* state was one of non-attachment to the world, despite their continuing *physical* presence within it. In the words of one, "After turning everything over to my son, I said to myself, 'Let me leave everything and take *sannyas* [Renunciation].' Yes, even while continuing to live at home, it is as if I am in the Renouncer stage of life." Thus, while for most aging Hindus the extreme course of complete physical withdrawal from the world and its inhabitants is hardly either attractive or feasible, the knowledge that detachment from worldly concerns is required for spiritual advancement has distinct consequences for the kind of attitude they attempt to cultivate in contemplating life's end.

In trying to understand the basis for the characteristic Hindu approach toward aging and death it is important not to ignore the influence of the material and social environments in which they live. Death is a more familiar event for Indians than it is for us, both because mortality rates are somewhat higher than ours and because most deaths occur at home rather than in the hospital or nursing home. There is in Hindu society a familiar, "hands-on" relationship to dying and death that is minimally mediated by specialist professionals. Most adults have had, more than once, the experience of watching over a loved one in the throes of death, often a drawn out and painful passing. They have washed and prepared corpses for their final rites. Men have helped carry funeral biers to the cremation ground and have watched as they burned. They have ignited the funeral pyres of their deceased parents and, at the prescribed moment, cracked open their skulls with a wooden staff to release their vital breath. They have personally gathered together the ashes and bone fragments to dispose of them in the religiously prescribed manner.

In Indian society death is also spoken about more openly than it is in ours. Old men and women may often be heard to state quite cheerfully that they are ready to welcome death at any time, that they have lived long and satisfying lives and are prepared for the end. Doubtless they talk this way not only because it is considered culturally appropriate to cultivate equanimity in the prospect of death, but because the very act of repeatedly speaking of it helps them to achieve that state. In the same vein, a vigorous woman in her fifties described to me how once, after the death of a close relative, she had secretly followed the male-only funeral procession to the cremation ground and forced herself to watch for several hours the fiery destruction of the body. This experience, she maintained, helped her to come to terms with the prospect of her own eventual death.

An older man or woman who follows the culture's normative guidelines for appropriate behavior in old age—allowing adult children to run their own lives and manage their household without interference—reaps clear personal benefits. If a person does become incapacitated, he (or she) is much more likely to be cared for willingly and well if he has already developed good relationships with his sons and daughters-in-law. Most old people live in the same household with these family members and it is this younger generation who will take on the care of an aging invalid. In India the retirement or nursing home is almost unknown, and old people, particularly in rural areas, rarely use hospital facilities. Aside from practical limitations on access to modern medical care, old age and its afflictions are typically held to be simply part of the nature of things—and because they are incurable it is futile to seek treatment. Furthermore, if one goes to the hospital one risks the awful possibility of dying away from home and family.

What message does this review of the Hindu art of dying have for us? Clearly there would be little point in proposing our wholesale adoption of a set of alien cosmological notions and social norms. However, there are real lessons to be learned from Indian openness to speaking about death and to entering into a dialogue with loved ones about the prospect of their own deaths. There is also a lesson to be learned from the way that Hindus situate death for the old in the milieu of the home and family rather than that of the medical institution with its specialist caregivers. Finally, we may learn from the Hindu's conscious recognition and acceptance of his own mortality and his consequent striving to prepare for a good death. None of these lessons, nor the recommendations to which they lead, are new—all have been discussed and debated for years by scholars, medical practitioners, and the general public. But my discussion of a living culture in which these benefits are realized may serve to further support the many voices that today call for a new approach to how we die in America.

Notes

1. It should be pointed out that all Indians are not Hindu. Over 10 percent are Muslim, and there are significant adherents to Christianity and other religions as well. Many non-Hindu Indians share the overall cognitive orientation toward aging and death that I describe here, but my specific focus is on the use Hindus make of their own religious, cosmological and normative concepts as they grow older and face the prospect of their own mortality.

2. See Keyes and Daniel (1983) for a number of useful essays on popular understandings of this concept in various regions of India and southeast Asia. Another excellent collection of papers focusing on Hindu textual traditions is O'Flaherty 1980.

3. Shrinivas Tilak (1989, 15–51) provides a good historical overview of the development over time of the life course model in the Hindu textual tradition. For a more technical discussion, see Olivelle 1993.

4. The models provided in the texts apply explicitly to the male life course. Woman appears only as her husband's companion and helpmate. When he enters the fourth *ashrama* and renounces the world, his bond with her is one of those that he severs. Among the people I studied, however, a three- or four-stage model of the life course was commonly used to frame discourse about women's lives as well.

5. For elaboration of this point and further information about attitudes toward aging and death in this community, see Vatuk 1990.

References

Doniger, W., trans. 1991. *The laws of Manu*. London: Penguin Books.

Hiebert, P. 1981. Old age in a south Indian village. In *Other ways of growing old*, ed. P. T. Amoss and S. Harrell. Stanford, Calif.: Stanford University Press.

Keyes, C. F., and E. V. Daniel, eds. 1983. *Karma: An anthropological inquiry*. Berkeley: University of California Press.

Madan, T. N. 1988. *Non-renunciation: Themes and interpretations of Hindu culture*. Delhi: Oxford University Press.

O'Flaherty, W. D., ed. 1980. *Karma and rebirth in classical Indian traditions*. Berkeley: University of California Press.

Olivelle, P. 1993. *The asrama system: The history and hermeneutics of a religious institution*. New York: Oxford University Press.

Parry, J. 1982. Sacrificial death and the necrophagous ascetic. In *Death and the regeneration of life*, ed. M. Bloch and J. Parry. Cambridge, Eng.: Cambridge University Press.

———. 1994. *Death in Banaras*. Cambridge, Eng.: Cambridge University Press.

Tilak, S. 1989. *Religion and aging in the Indian tradition*. Albany: State University of New York Press.

Vatuk, S. 1990. "To be a burden on others": Dependency anxiety among the elderly in India. In *Divine passions: The social construction of emotion in India*, ed. O. Lynch. Berkeley: University of California Press.

Chapter 14

Reflections on Mortality from a Jewish Perspective

James E. Ponet

F rom beginning to end the Hebrew Scriptures are saturated with the consciousness of mortality. Time and limitation hang over the Genesis narrative of Creation, which culminates, significantly, not with the creation of humanity on the sixth day, but rather with a grand cessation of activity on the seventh. "The heaven and earth were finished, and all their array. On the seventh day God *finished* the work that He had been doing, and He *ceased* on the seventh day from all the work that He had done. And God *blessed* the seventh day and *declared it holy*, because on it God ceased from all the work of creation that He had done" (Gn 2:1–3).

Notice the themes of completion and cessation, asserted by the use of two separate verbs, and the conjunction of these ideas with the notion of blessing and sanctity. The fulfillment of creation, it turns out, is rest; we are left with the strange metaphor of an all powerful Creator who, having ordered a universe into existence, now stands as it were to the side and watches it—God as birdwatcher or stargazer.

How did God feel in the first moments after Creation? What consciousness accompanied the Lord's Sabbath observance? This genre of question is both articulated and addressed in the post-Biblical Midrashic literature. A fourth-century commentary on the Book of Genesis, *Bereshit Rabba*, compares God to the father of a bride gazing upon his daughter as she stands under the wedding canopy. As he looks at her he thinks, "My daughter would that you could always be as beautiful as you are today." Similarly God gazes wistfully at creation and thinks, "My world! My world! Would that you could always be as beautiful to Me as you are at this moment" (*Bereshit Rabba* 9:4).

But if decay, decomposition, and destruction are in fact natural to the Biblical world view, how is one to understand the captivating etiology of death offered in the Garden of Eden passages in Genesis chapters 2 and 3?

If in fact death was built into the constitution of reality by the Creator's original fiat, how is one to understand God's declaration to Adam at Genesis 2:16–17: "Of every tree of the garden you are free to eat, but from the tree of the knowledge of good and evil, you shall not eat; for on the day you eat of it you will surely die." And how is one to understand God's angry proclamation of mortality at 3:17–19? "Because you did as your wife said and ate of the tree about which I commanded you, 'You shall not eat of it,' the earth shall be cursed because of you. By toil you shall eat of it all the days of your life: thorns and thistles shall it sprout for you. But your food shall be the grasses of the field; by the sweat of your brow shall you get bread to eat, until you return to the earth—for from it were you taken. For dust you are, and to dust you shall return."

Is death then punishment, the product of Adam's disobedience, or is death rather part and parcel of the human condition? Upon scrutiny one is forced to admit that the Genesis death narratives are murky. Rather than offer a clear answer to the great question, "Why do people die?" these texts in fact sow seeds of perplexity that for millennia have been harvested in the extensive literature responding to the reality of finitude.

PHILOSOPHICAL AND MYSTICAL RESPONSES

The philosophical sensibility within Judaism early on was reconciled to the inevitability of death and even strove to create a positive acceptance of death. Thus a fourth-century Midrash records that in the margins of his own Torah scroll Rebbe Meir wrote that Genesis 1:31—which reads, "And God saw all that He had created and behold it was *tov m'od*, very good"—should be read, "And God saw all that He had created and behold *tov mot*, death is good" (*Bereshit Rabba* 9:5). Maimonides incorporated this Midrash into his twelfth-century philosophical magnum opus, *The Guide of the Perplexed*, where he wrote: "Even the existence of this inferior matter, whose manner of being it is to be a concomitant of privation entailing death and all evils, all this is also *good* in view of the perpetuity of generation and the permanence of being through succession" (*Guide* 3:10).

One disciple of Maimonides, Biblical commentator Rabbi David Kimhi—who died in Provence in 1235, thirty years after Maimonides died in Egypt—read Genesis 2:17, "But from the tree of the knowledge of good and evil you shall not eat for on the day you eat from it you will surely die," to mean "On the day you eat from it, it will be decreed that you shall die sooner than you would have otherwise" (Kimhi, 1926). Adam would have lived a thousand years; instead he died at age 930.

The mystical sensibility in Judaism, on the other hand, reads in the Genesis texts that humanity was created to live forever and that the arrival of death was a tragic interruption that must somehow, someday be over-come. Thus the thirteenth-century Spanish jurist, commentator, and kab-balist Rabbi Moses Nachmanides (d. 1270) reads Genesis 2:17, "But from the tree of the knowledge of good and evil you shall not eat for on the day you eat from it you will surely die," as teaching that Adam became mortal only after his disobedient consumption of fruit from that tree. A physician like Maimonides, Nachmanides insisted that the art of medicine was primi-tive compared to the divine science of healing by faith, for the human being is not merely natural. "Know that only faithless people who believe the world exists by necessity hold that the body is necessarily subject to corrup-tion. But according to the faithful who hold that the world was created by the will of God, a human life can last forever so long as God wills it" (Ramban 1973; also at Lv 26:11). For the mystics, access to the will of God offers the possibility of overcoming the terms of life in the present. For the philosophers mortality cannot be overcome, but with the acquisition of wisdom it can be endured. Between these points of view a war of sensibility rages.

Although mortal, Biblical Adam lived 930 years. A few generations later, Methusaleh achieved 960 years. The Book of Genesis records the shrinking of life spans. Abraham reached 175 although Sarah only 127. Isaac reached 180, but Jacob did not reach 150. Tired, old Jacob (Gn 47:7–11), in a gesture that suggests the onset of senescence, greets Pharaoh for the first time, and in response to the potentate's question, "How old are you?" answers, "The years of my sojourn [on earth] are one hundred and thirty. Few and hard have been the years of my life, nor do they come up to the life span of my fathers during their sojourns."

THE DEATH OF MOSES

It is however the six score years of Moses that set the Bible's standard for humanity. Thus the Talmud reports that Rabbi Yochanan ben Zakkai and Rabbi Akiva both lived 120 years. And on this basis there developed the tradition of wishing someone a happy birthday by saying, "May you live to a hundred and twenty." The Book of Deuteronomy makes it clear that Moses' death was not the result of gradual erosion of his faculties, the culmination of a process of illness and loss; rather "his eyes were un-dimmed and his vigor unabated." Moses responded, as it were, to the divine summons "ascend this mountain and die" (Dt 32:50) simply because it was time. The Five Books that begin with Creation find their culmina-tion here in the death of Moses.

Moses standing atop Mount Nebo gazing wistfully across the Jordan into the land that he will never enter—this is the signature of the Torah.

Not death itself, but incompletion haunts the man who has reached his life's limit. The Bible calls Psalm 90 "the Prayer of Moses," for in it these words appear: "You return man to dust. You decreed, 'Return you mortals.' For in Your sight a thousand years are like yesterday that has past, like a watch of the night. You engulf men in sleep; at daybreak they are like grass that renews itself; at daybreak it flourishes anew, by dusk it withers and dries up. . . . The span of our life is seventy years, or, given the strength, eighty years; but the best of them are trouble and sorrow. . . . Teach us to number our days that we may obtain a wise heart."

Moses' death is dignified, simple, paradigmatic. The text says that God buried him in a valley opposite Jericho in a place no one knows. Only once in Deuteronomy is there a suggestion that Moses sought to resist the command to die. "'Lord God, You have just begun to show your servant Your unparalleled greatness and might. . . . Let me cross over so that I may see the good land which is on the other side of the Jordan.' . . . But the Lord had became angry with me because of you and refused to listen to me. And the Lord said to me, 'This is enough for you. Speak to Me no further about this. Ascend the mountain and lift your eyes west, north, south, and east—but you shall not cross this Jordan'" (Dt 3:24–27).

Biblical Moses ultimately accepts the divine decree with grace, but the Moses of Midrash stages a grand struggle with death. We might say that Biblical Moses dies a good death in a hospice while Midrashic Moses is hooked to a vast array of life-support mechanisms that doom him to a protracted struggle with the inevitable. Consider the Deuteronomic description of Moses' death: "Moses went up from the steppes of Moab to Mount Nebo, to the summit of Pisgah, opposite Jericho, and the Lord showed him the whole land. . . . And the Lord said to him, 'This is the land of which I swore to Abraham, Isaac and Jacob, "I will assign it to your offspring." I have let you see it with your own eyes, but you shall not cross there.' So Moses the servant of God died there in the land of Moab, at the command of the Lord" (Dt 34:1–4).

Compare this simple tale of obedience with the following segment from a tenth-century Midrashic compendium known as *Midrash P'tirat Moshe* (The Midrash of the death of Moses):

> When the day for Moses our teacher, may he rest in peace, came to depart the world, the Holy One Blessed be He said to him, "Your days have drawn near to die" (Dt 31:14). Moses replied, "Master of the Universe, after all the work that I have done, You say that I should die. 'I will not die but will live and recount the glory of God'" (Ps 118:17).
> The Holy Blessed be He said to him, "Enough for you. You come this far and

no further. Call Joshua so that I may give him his orders." He responded, "Master of the Universe, why must I die? If it is for the sake of Joshua's honor, let Joshua take over and I will give up my responsibilities." The Holy One Blessed be He said to him, "You will treat him the way he has treated you?" He answered, "Yes."

Moses began to walk behind Joshua and to call him Rabbi Joshua. Joshua became very frightened and cried out to him, "Me, you call Rabbi?!" Moses our teacher, may he rest in peace, said to Joshua, "Do you want me to live and not die?" He answered, "Yes." He said to him, "Isn't it good for you that I don't die like this? If any part of the job overwhelms you, I will instruct you. But understand that I shall live and that I will treat you the way you used to treat me." Joshua replied to Moses our teacher, may he rest in peace, "Whatever you decree upon me I will accept just so that I may continue to see your face."

So Moses our teacher, may he rest in peace, proceeded to exalt Joshua the way Joshua had previously exalted him. When they entered the tent of meeting the pillar of cloud descended . . . between Moses and Joshua, with Joshua inside and Moses our teacher, may he rest in peace, outside. But when he saw what had happened, he said, "Better a hundred deaths than one moment of envy."

Moses then began to appeal his sentence before God. He said to Him, "Master of the Universe, what sin have I committed that I should die?" The Holy One Blessed be He answered him, "Because of the sin of Adam . . . you must die." He replied, "Master of the Universe, was it for naught that my feet entered the cloud of the divine presence, and for naught that I ran like a horse before Your children?" He answered, "I have already sentenced humanity to die."

He said to him, "Master of the Universe, You gave Adam but a single simple commandment and he transgressed it. But I have not transgressed." He answered, "Abraham sanctified My Name in the world yet he died. . . ." He said to him, "Master of the Universe, will not people say that if God had not found evil things in Moses He never would have forced him from the world?" He answered, "I already wrote in My Torah, 'Never again did there arise in Israel a prophet like Moses—whom the Lord singled out face to face. . . ' " (Dt 34:10). "Maybe they will say that in my youth I obeyed You but in my old age I rebelled." "I already wrote that you did not sanctify Me [at the waters of Meribath-Kadesh in the wilderness of Zin]" (Dt 32:51).

He said to Him, "Master of the Universe, let me enter the land of Israel, live there for two or three years, and then I will die."

"I have decreed that You shall not enter there."

"If I cannot enter in my life, let me at least enter in my death."

"No!"

He said to Him, "Master of the Universe, why is all this anger directed at me?"

Although he must ultimately succumb, Moses disdains all of God's arguments and dismisses all of God's messengers. He dies alone, tradition teaches, with God's kiss on his lips (B. Talmud, Moed Katan 28A). Note that in structuring the dialogue between God and Moses the author of *Midrash P'tirat Moshe* does not resort to the argument for reward after death even though it was available to him. It is significant that Moses does not renounce this world in order to gain a greater prominence in the next. Rather, his loss is absolute. He had sought entrance to a land from which he was barred, the dark truth of all death.

LIVING WITH DEATH

Then what strategies, if any, does Judaism provide for reconciling mortals to their mortality? The simplest strategy is the appropriation of one's death as a deserved punishment. Happy the mortal who can die with the sense of having earned mortality. Clearly Midrashic Moses was incapable of apprehending his own death in this manner, even though the Bible offers the explanation of his having failed to sanctify God's Name at Meribath-Kadesh. If every death cannot be construed as punishment, still it is possible, in the spirit of "visiting the sins of the fathers upon the children" (Ex 20), to construe each death as a derivative punishment, yet another echo of Adam's betrayal. But this thought too carried no conviction for Midrashic Moses.

Perhaps a more subtle strategem is the construal of death as expiation or atonement. "May my death be an atonement for all of my sins." According to the Talmud, these words are to be extracted if possible from the criminal convicted of a capital offense in the moments before execution (B. Talmud, Sanhedrin 43A); they are also offered as part of the voluntary liturgy of confession on one's deathbed. If one can accept the judgment of Ecclesiastes, "There is not a just man upon the earth who does good and does not sin" (7:20), and on this basis come to recognize one's deepest human failures, one may then possibly arrive at the conclusion that some sins can only be overturned, sweetened, or transformed by the mysterious sacrifice of death (B. Talmud, Yoma 86A, and Maimonides, *Laws of Repentance* 1:4).

Every deathbed might then be understood as a kind of sacrificial altar. In dying one would become simultaneously a priest, a supplicant, and an offering. In this sense each death becomes an act of *kiddush hashem,* a heroic expression of total commitment, a conscious act of giving oneself away, a kind of martyrdom. According to the expiation theory of death, dying in full consciousness can be a way of achieving full reconciliation with the Source of Life from which one necessarily becomes alienated during one's life.

Jewish tradition knows to distinguish a good death—that is, a fast death after the age of eighty—from a bad death (B. Talmud, Moed Katan 28A). It does not, however, assert that death is good. Jewish law establishes mourning as a mandatory response on the part of the survivors. After his two sons, Nadav and Avihu, died, the Book of Leviticus (9:24ff.) recounts that Aharon, Moses' brother, the High Priest of Israel, did not eat the communal sin offering as was his official responsibility. His apparent neglect of his office earned him a reproach from Moses to which Aharon fetchingly responded, "Such things have befallen me that had I eaten the sin offering today, would it have been good in God's eyes?" (10:19).

From this encounter between the brothers, the Talmud establishes the obligation to mourn. (B. Talmud Zevakhim 101A, Maimonides, *Laws of Entering the Temple,* 2:6–9, and *Laws of Mourning* 1:1.) It says that Moses himself, who initially did not recognize the need—or remember the legal obligation—to mourn, ordained the mourning period of seven days known as *shiva.* The Talmudic Sages expanded that unit to thirty days known as *shloshim.* But while the obligation to mourn is clear, the nature of mourning remains unresolved. Is mourning essentially a concession to human weakness, a permission to express anger and pain at life's injustice? Or is mourning more aptly construed as a duty owed the departed, a refusal to give death victory over one whose life was so precious? Is mourning for the survivors or for the deceased? Does it reflect human weakness or human strength, brokenness or integrity?

In the act of mourning, Jewish tradition attempts both to acknowledge and to deny death. Thus the Pentateuch ends with God himself burying Moses and with God offering Moses' eulogy: "Never again did there arise in Israel a prophet like Moses—whom the Lord singled out, face to face, for the various signs and portents that the Lord sent him to display in the land of Egypt, against Pharaoh and all his courtiers and his whole country, and for all the great might and awesome power that Moses displayed before all Israel" (Dt 34:10–12).

These words end the Torah. The Five Books of Moses begin with a Creation narrative that features a God who rests on the seventh day, and they end with a death narrative that features a God who buries and eulogizes His creation. God the Creator is God the mourner.

References

B. *Talmud.* 1936. London: Soncino Press.
Kimhi, D. 1926– . *The commentary of David Kimhi on Isaiah . . . with his allegorical commentary on Genesis.* Ed. L. Finkelstein. New York: Columbia University Press.

Maimonides. 1963. *Guide of the perplexed.* Trans. Shlomo Pines. Chicago: University of Chicago Press.

———. *Laws of entering the temple.* From Mishneh Torah, Book of Worship.

———. *Laws of mourning.* From Mishneh Torah, Book of Judges.

———. *Laws of repentance.* From Mishneh Torah, Book of Knowledge.

The Midrash Rabbah. 1977. New York: Soncino Press.

Ramban (Nachmanides). 1973. *Commentary on the Torah.* Trans. C. B. Chavel. New York: Shilo.

Tanakh: A new translation of The Holy Scriptures according to the traditional Hebrew text. 1965. New York: Jewish Publication Society.

Chapter 15

Catholic Theology's Main Thoughts on Death

Harald Wagner

The universality of death is one of the main affirmations of Catholic faith. Faith teaches that all human beings are subject to the law of death and that all will, in fact, die. Though this proposition seems to be knowable through a process of empirical deduction, because of its source in divine revelation it possesses an entirely different character from the identical statement based upon human experience. Holy Scripture says: All human beings are sinners, therefore all human beings die. Thus, death is one of the necessary or essential features of human existence; it will never be possible to abolish death. Even if there is a natural explanation for the necessity and universality of death (whether chemical or medical), it still has to be said: All human beings die because all are sinners.

The dogma of the universality of death describes the phenomenon of death from the outside. A second proposition of faith comes closer to the essence of death. The traditional formulation describes death as the separation of body and soul. Christian faith, however, is not dualistic. It is the human being as a whole who dies. In death, something happens to each person as a whole. Since the soul is united to the body essentially, it must clearly have some relationship to the body after death (or better: it must clearly have some relationship to that whole of which the body is a part, to the material universal). The description of death as a separation of body and soul leaves room for further philosophical and theological distinctions. This proposition affirms that with bodily death the human state of pilgrimage (to employ the usual theological expression) comes to a definite end. This doctrine of faith involves taking this earthly life with radical seriousness. Human life is suspended between a beginning and an end. There is no eternal return of all things; there is only history, happening once and for all. Christian faith does not allow for the migration of souls.

WHAT DOES *ARS MORIENDI* MEAN?

As I pointed out at the beginning, the Christian faith teaches the universality of death. Death is a part of human life. "Man is," the German philosopher Martin Heidegger has said, "the being towards death." Only when I understand what death is can I understand what life is. From this, each person should draw the logical conclusions concerning his or her own personal death and his or her own dealings with dying and death in his or her own life. Our ancestors did this. They developed their own *ars moriendi* [on the craft of dying]. Just as at that time one learned the art of loving (*ars amandi*) and the art of hunting (*ars venandi*), so too, one also wanted to learn how one might die correctly. Perhaps a reconsideration of the *ars moriendi* might once again be of use to all of us in accepting the existential challenge of death and dying.

In the late Middle Ages, works related to *ars moriendi* developed as a special literary genre. Nearly all of the authors were clergy. Among these handbooks, two were especially famous: the *Ars moriendi* (c. 1450–60) of the chancellor of Paris, Jean Gerson, and the *Speculum artis bene moriendi* (c. 1452), whose author we have not determined. All were handbooks intended to be an aid to pastors and their assistants on how they were to behave at the sickbed and deathbed. It was important that clergy know what happens to the dying, what the dying person experiences. The handbooks on *ars moriendi* formed a kind of dogma concerning dying.

The structure and contents of these handbooks on death vary. One can, nonetheless, find common elements in them. At the beginning are always considerations concerning the nature of death. Then follows a list of questions that the priest should ask the dying person, in order to assure that he or she assumes the correct attitude toward death. The priest asks the dying person, for example, whether he seeks forgiveness of sins from God; whether she is conscious of unforgiven mortal sins; whether he wishes to return something he has stolen; whether she has forgiven those who have insulted her. These handbooks also contain prayers to be said with the dying person. Those prayers speak of submission to God's will, patient endurance of suffering and death, grateful acknowledgment of God's gifts in this life, and perfect devotion to God.

Of special interest is the section containing *observationes* (observations). These are various aids and instructions for the one keeping company with the dying person. It explains the stages through which the dying person passes: despair, hope, impatience, submission to God's will. In this context, Elisabeth Kübler-Ross comes to mind. The companion of the dying person is given practical advice as to what to do: read aloud, ask questions, take the dying person's mind off the cares of this world, and, if need be, keep the family away.

Some defining characteristics of these handbooks might be of particular import to us. First, their basic concern is the human. The pastor tries to do the right thing for the person who finds him- or herself in the unique situation of dying. Upon looking back, the dying person should put in order that which has been left in disorder in his or her life. The dying person should pass through the experience of dying quietly and calmly. He or she is to be consoled in his or her suffering. One author of an *ars moriendi* states that the companion to the dying person should at least *consolatorias effundere lacrymas* (shed tears of sympathy). Christian belief guides and is interwoven with this care for the dying—the person in his or her present condition is the object of all-inclusive care.

A second central concern of these handbooks is truth. The person who has lived life consciously will be able to die in peace. That person has consistently recognized and understood the "messengers" of death: illness, farewells, symptoms of aging. Even if that person has not become better acquainted with these, nevertheless he or she should not deceive him- or herself shortly before dying. The person who is ill should be aware of his or her condition. That person's vision should be directed toward Christ, who says, "I am the Way, the Truth, and the Life." To make the approach to the truth of death easier, this literature gives an important piece of advice: Tell the person, while he or she is still healthy, to find a friend (called *amicus aegroti* [friend of the sick] or simply *amicus*) to talk to about death and dying and to be present when one is dying.

Third, death as a break in human existence is taken seriously. None can wish himself dead when the time for this death has not yet arrived. Everyone who can should help through craft and study (*arte et studio*) to lengthen human life. It is a sin to reject a physician's help. On the other hand, death belongs to the totality of life. Therefore it should be passed through and suffered consciously.

ARS MORIENDI FOR TODAY

It is necessary for us to confront the fact of death again and again, for only those who have understood death understand life. Therefore we all need to deal inwardly and outwardly with this fact. I am thinking first of all of very practical things.

Practice in dying begins with clearing out, with throwing out and getting rid of all which is an encumbrance. It is a proven exemplary practice to go through one's house every five years or so and get rid of everything that has no more value. One must be rigorous in doing this. "For where your treasure is, there will your heart be also" (Mt 6:21, RSV). Look at all your "treasures" very carefully and imagine being a relative who must put all of this into order and break it up after your death. This exercise has a sobering effect and makes getting rid of things much easier. Giving things away is another form of freeing oneself from those things that weigh one down. Some things are much too valuable simply to throw away. By giving them away, one can make others happy.

It is also important to write a last will and testament early on, in order to determine what will happen to that which one leaves behind. In doing so, we detach ourselves inwardly from that which we possess. Inwardly then, we have already given it away. We learn how to give away, how to detach ourselves, as an attitude toward our external lives. We become persons who "have as though they did not have" (1 Cor 7:30).

It is very difficult for people today to come to the decision that they should or must develop their own *ars moriendi* for themselves. The ground for this has hardly been prepared in our time. I believe that everyone who is in a position to do so must seek to ensure that the dual topic of dying and death is treated in schools. Only then will one become sensitized to one's own susceptibility to death. Students should learn and realize far more than has been the case that human beings are mortal. Everyone grows older; each person's supply of life is limited. Educators can communicate to children a knowledge of death that corresponds to reality. This is to be done as a help toward living, toward forming one's own life in view of this fact.

Children and young people should not only learn what it means to be mortal, however. They should become acquainted with the various manners of dying—physical and social death, violent and natural death. They should learn how to interpret death. Christians should learn the Christian interpretation of death. Those who take death seriously will have become sensitized to the uniqueness and dignity of humankind.

I would therefore plead for an extendable "thanagogic," which will not be confined to the school framework, though it has a very special place there. It is not to be restricted to lessons in religion. School is the place where youth are prepared for life; this important purpose must be fulfilled there.

Let us call to mind again that the *Ars moriendi* was a help for pastors in their care of the dying. This task remains important today. Indeed, it is becoming ever more important. Not only pastors, but also physicians, nurses, and all those who are professionally concerned with the sick and dying must once again learn how to deal appropriately with the dying. Furthermore, everyone must learn this art, as everyone will at one time or another be confronted with death. At one time or another, everyone is "the next of kin." *The Dying Need Solidarity* is the title of a book Torsten Kruse and I wrote. Why do the dying need solidarity? Why must we care for them in a special way? In dealing with the dying we can learn a great deal about our own death and to understand the paradox: dying is a phase of human living, part of the biography of human life.

By way of conclusion, let me offer some observations. Without death, life would be boring: everything would be indifferent, alike, repeatable, susceptible to deferral. The philosopher W. Kaufmann has said, "one leads a better life when one has made a rendezvous with death." The proximity of death gives life depth. Indeed, I would question whether human beings would become more human if medicine succeeded in prolonging life even longer. Life would become superficial if it did not face the limits death places on it: the sense of responsibility would be lost. Were there no death, one could begin anew anytime. Life would lose its direction. It is for all these reasons that an *ars moriendi* is so important for our time.

Chapter 16

The Law of the Spirits: Chinese Popular Beliefs

Valerie Hansen

The Chinese were not sure what happened after death. Some Buddhist sects promised rebirth in a paradise and Daoism, immortality to a chosen few. Still, the majority of the dead, it was thought, went to an underworld. There they retained the power to influence events on earth. If they wanted to hurt the living they could play tricks, cause illness, provoke misfortune, or even bring death. Some of the deceased performed miracles and came to be worshipped as gods. The Chinese feared the dead, but they believed that they adhered to their own laws. These three readings from the eleventh and twelfth centuries show how the living used the law of the spirits to protect themselves from the dangers posed by the dead.

The first document in this selection is a model tomb contract from *The New Book of Earth Patterns,* a government manual for siting graves initially published in 1071. Starting in the first century A.D., if not earlier, and continuing through to the twentieth century, some Chinese buried tomb contracts with the dead. Mimicking this-worldly contracts for the purchase of land, these contracts recorded the purchase of a grave plot from the earth gods. Tomb contracts were intended to ward off the dangers that resulted from penetrating deep into the earth to dig a grave. The practice seems to have peaked in the Song dynasty (960–1279), when the government paid for such contracts to be drawn up on behalf of dead officials (Tuo et al. 1977, 2909–10). Just after the Song had fallen, Zhou Mi (1232–1298) said: "Today when people make tombs they always use a certificate to buy land, made out of catalpa wood, on which they write in red, saying: 'Using 99,999 strings of cash, we buy a certain plot, and so forth.'" Nine was an auspicious number; hence the figure 99,999. The money in these contracts was not real money, but spirit money (facsimiles of real money) that could be burnt. Not all contracts were written on catalpa wood. Hundreds of lead and stone tomb contracts have been excavated, and presumably more were written on cheaper materials, like paper or wood, that have since decayed.

The New Book of Earth Patterns was written at imperial order by a team of scholars, headed by Wang Zhu, who examined preexisting ritual manuals and then compiled this book. This manual was intended for official use, but commoners also consulted it, Wang Zhu tells us. In the section about tomb contracts, *The New Book of Earth Patterns* cites *The Spirit Code (Guilü)* to say that burial without using a tomb contract is tantamount to wrongful burial and very unlucky. The idea of a law code for spirits raises interesting issues: Why should spirits have a law code? Is it written down? What is its relation to human law? These questions are not easily answered, but the widespread use of tomb contracts reveals that many people believed (or hoped) that the spirits of the dead could be bound by contracts. The similarity of the contracts to this-worldly contracts also suggests that they thought the law of the spirits resembled earthly law.

Because *The New Book of Earth Patterns* spells out the many steps of an official funeral ritual, it describes the ritual context in which tomb contracts were used. The manual specifies that any official with the posthumous rank of lord or marquis and below (or any commoners paying for their own funerals) should have two iron contracts: one was to be placed in the temporary above-ground funeral structure and the other, buried in front of the coffin. Then a prayer is said. Once the prayer is completed, the two copies of the contract are held together, and the characters for agreement (*hetong*) are written on the seam where the two join. Borrowed from real life, this practice ensured that either the buyer or seller could check the authenticity of a contract by matching it with their copy to see if the characters met exactly. If they did, then the contract was authentic, and the signatories were bound to honor it. If they did not, it was a forgery. At the end of the funeral, the participants took the iron contract in the temporary funeral structure and buried it in the ground. That was the gods' copy. The one at the foot of the coffin was for the master of the tomb, the dead official. He needed to have his copy with him in case he had a dispute in the underworld with the spirits of the dead about his ownership of his funeral plot.

The text of the model contract follows contemporary land contracts very closely. It gives the date of the transaction—here the date of the funeral— and the name of the buyer, the dead person, without naming the seller, the lord of the earth. As was true of land contracts, the dimensions of the plot are given in two ways: on a grid with the north-south and east-west axes, and by naming the neighbors, who were the animals who watched over the four directions. The price was the usual 99,999 strings of cash as well as offerings of five-colored paper. The contract then specifies the consequences if the contract is violated: any spirits who return from the dead (read: to bother the deceased or his living kin) will be tied up and handed over to the earl of the rivers. Like a land contract, the contract contains a clause saying it will take effect once the money and land have been exchanged, which, in this case, must mean when the paper money is burned at the funeral and the body interred. The contract ends with the names of the witnesses, who can serve as intermediaries should any disputes occur, and the names of the guarantors, who will make good the buyer's price should he fail to come up with the money. The mystical identities of the neighbors, witnesses, and guarantors mark this as a tomb contract. After the end of the contract comes an amendment specifically prohibiting the former occupants of the grave plot from approaching the dead. Only if they stay ten thousand *li* away[1] can the deceased and his kin enjoy peace and good fortune. The contract ends by invoking the statutes and edicts of Nüqing, the emissary of the Five Emperors of the directions (north, south, east, west, and middle). These statutes and edicts are part of the spirit law code.

Of fifteen excavated contracts I have found that follow the model given in *The New Book of Earth Patterns,* eleven date to the Song dynasty. They show a surprising geographic range, which testifies to the wide circulation the manual enjoyed: to the west, from Xinjiang and Sichuan; to the north, from Shanxi and Shaanxi; in central China, from Hebei, Henan, Hubei, and Anhui: and to the southeast, from Jiangsu, Zhejiang, Jiangxi, and Fujian. Most of these tombs contain lavish grave goods, suggesting that the people who used this text were well-off.

The text of *The New Book of Earth Patterns* does not explicitly mention the dangers the spirits of the dead pose to the newly dead or his living kin, but another text found in a tomb in southeast China, Jiangxi, does. The text is written on the eight-sided body of a cedar figure, which had a carved human head with ears, eyes, mouth, and nose. Dated 1090, the figure was found in the tomb of the eighth daughter of the Yi family, a woman from an important local family (according to her biography, which is only partially quoted in the excavation report). She was interred in a wood coffin enclosed in a stone coffin. With her were buried two pottery vases, a pottery figure, her biography carved on a stone plaque, porcelain plates, wooden combs, iron scissors, an iron knife, an iron stick, a copper mirror, a large ax, and some items of relatively high quality: a silver comb, two silver bracelets, and a pair of gold earrings. Clearly, this was an expensive burial.

This text presumes a different relationship with the spirits of the dead than does *The New Book of Earth Patterns.* Here there is no contract with the lord of the earth for the purchase of the grave. Instead a cedar figure is deputed by those who preside over the world of the dead to prevent any lawsuits against the dead woman's family. The text repeats the same phrases over and over in its list of who cannot be summoned or sued by those in the middle of the earth—that is, by the spirits of the dead. It does not say what such a summons would result in, but presumably the people mentioned in the text—the dead woman's children, husband, siblings, family, and in-laws—would suffer some kind of misfortune or even death. Those in the middle of the earth also have the power to bring epidemics. And they can summon fields, silkworms, farm animals, and trees, and so cause havoc on people's farms. Because this text is designed to protect the dead and their descendants, its repetitious phrasing takes on the quality of an incantation. The cedar figure is the subterranean equivalent of a henchman whose job it is to prevent anyone from serving his mistress with a court summons.

The final text in this selection shows what happens when the underworld court issues a summons. It is an anecdote from a collection called *The Record of the Listener (Yijianzhi)*.[2] From 1157 to 1202, an official named Hong Mai transcribed thousands of strange and unusual tales. Many of these tales, like the one translated here, are about people who visit the netherworld and come back. The Chinese word for death, *si,* means both to faint and to lose consciousness; many people had unusual visions when they fainted, which they recounted on awaking. The events and miracles Hong Mai describes may defy belief, but these were the kinds of stories circulating in twelfth-century China, and Hong Mai often, as here, gives the name of the person who told him the anecdote. This source, then, can provide insight into the beliefs of poorer people in the Song dynasty, people who could not afford elaborate burials like those specified in *The New Book of Earth Patterns* or like that of the eighth daughter of the Yi family.

The anecdote begins with the facts of the case: the debtor Mr. Lin bribed the clerks in the local court to frame the lender, Registrar Xia. The one person willing to speak out on Registrar Xia's behalf is Liu Yuan Balang. In his eloquent refusal to be bought off by Mr. Lin's underlings, he raises the possibility of a court in the underworld where wrongs can be righted. Registrar Xia then dies, after instructing his sons to bury all the relevant documents concerning Mr. Lin's unpaid debt, because he plans to sue in the underworld court. A month later Mr. Lin's eight underlings die, and Liu Yuan Balang has a premonition that he is going to be summoned to testify. Because he is convinced of his innocence, he does not fear that he personally has to stand trial, so he assures his wife that he will return after two or three days. And he loses consciousness.

The narrative resumes when he wakes up. He has indeed been summoned to the netherworld court to serve as a witness. When Liu Yuan Balang arrives, he sees that Registrar Xia has succeeded in his suit against Mr. Lin's eight underlings, whose necks are encased in a wooden frame called a *canque*. Liu's account reveals much about the workings of the netherworld court, which are similar but not identical to those of a human court. In this vision, the presiding official is the king of the netherworld, not an underworld district magistrate. As on earth, he is served by clerks, who keep records and guide the prisoners from place to place. On hearing Liu's account, the king awards him an extra ten years of life.

The king sits in judgment on the dead, who await their appearances before him in a kind of purgatory that Liu visits on his way out. There Liu sees people who have committed various offenses. They tell him they "borrowed" money, rent, and possessions, but in fact they stole them with no intent to return the goods. Some ask for money. Others ask their family members for merits; this reflects the Buddhist belief that merits accrued by one person for doing good deeds can be transferred to another. The king urges Liu to tell the living about his court, and then the runner who has accompanied Liu asks for a bribe. The always righteous Liu refuses, and he wakes up in this world when the clerk in the netherworld pushes him to the ground. The proof that he did indeed journey to the netherworld is two-fold: his false topknot lies dislodged on his pillow, and he lives for an extra decade past eighty. The story concludes with Hong Mai's explanation of how he heard it.

This anecdote is about justice. Registrar Xia is unable to obtain justice in human courts, but, as Liu Yuan Balang suspects, the underworld does have a court where wrongs can be righted. Many accounts of visits to the netherworld survive, and many tell of bureaucratic incompetence, of clerks who summon someone with an identical or a similar name by mistake. These people are then allowed to return to life. Strikingly, no one is ever punished in the subterranean court for a crime he or she did not commit. What about the real villain Mr. Lin? The account does not reveal his fate, and the reader knows only that Registrar Xia is able to sue the eight underlings. Mr. Lin may be punished after he dies when he is tried before the king. Or perhaps he has already been punished, but Liu simply does not see him because he was not party to the bribery attempt.

The story about Registrar Xia and Mr. Lin illustrates exactly what the people who used tomb contracts and the cedar figure feared. Registrar Xia may be dead, but he is still able to bring charges against the living in the underworld court. He causes not only the deaths of the eight underlings but also their continued suffering in the afterlife. Other spirits had the same power to sue in underworld courts. Digging a grave is dangerous:

one could unwittingly antagonize the previous owners who could claim title to the plot. That was why people used tomb contracts. That was not the only danger. Once someone went before the underworld court, a host of charges could be brought against the deceased and their descendants based on their previous conduct. It was in order to block those charges that the eighth daughter of the Yi family buried the cedar figure in her tomb.

The legalistic thinking in these three readings is striking. The model tomb contract in *The New Book of Earth Patterns* is just like a contract to purchase land. The cedar person is just like a henchman hired to prevent the issuing of summonses. And Registrar Xia encounters a court in the netherworld very much like the one in the human world—except that justice is done there. What kind of people would conceive of contracts with spirits, of spirit summonses, of a netherworld court? Surely only a people thoroughly familiar with the earthly legal system could envision such an afterlife.

Notes

I should like to thank Victor Mair, Liu Xinru, and Bao Weimin for their help with these translations and the late Anna Seidel for her many insights into the netherworld system of justice.

1. A *li* is about a third of a mile. Ten thousand *li* is a figure of speech that means a great distance.

2. For more about this book, see my *Changing Gods in Medieval China*, 17–23.

References

Hansen, V. 1990. *Changing gods in medieval China.* Princeton, N.J.: Princeton University Press.

Hong, M. 1981. *Yijian zhi.* Beijing: Zhonghua shuju, sec. "Zhiwu," chap. 5, p. 1086.

Peng, S., and Tang, C. 1980. "Jiangxi faxian jizuo BeiSong jinian mu." *Wenwu,* vol. 5.

Tuo, T., et al. 1977. *Songshi.* Beijing: Zhonghua shuju, chap. 77.

Wang, Z. n.d. *Dili xinshu.* Beijing library Jin ed., Chap. 14, p. 13a.

Zhou, M. n.d. *Guixin zashi* (Xuejin taoyuan ed.), chap. "bieji xia," pp. 7a–b.

Chapter 17

The Meaning of Death in Islam

Ira M. Lapidus

Muslim peoples today number some 900 million and represent a great variety of national, ethnic, language, tribal, and other communities. As Muslims they share certain common views about the nature of death and the afterlife, many common funeral and burial practices, and similar views about the significance of death for the living of life in this world. These views stem from the Qur'an, the book of revelations to the prophet Muhammad, the founder of Islam; the collections of the sayings of the prophet outside of the Qur'an (called hadith); and the commentaries of later scholars, jurists, Sufi mystics, theologians, and philosophers. This corpus of scriptures, commentary, and interpretation does not present a unified view about dying, death, and the afterlife, but for our purposes we will consider it a single canon or tradition.

Despite this shared religious heritage, there are still enormous variations in Muslim beliefs and practices about dying, death, funerals, burials, and commemorations, some of which derive from differences within the religious tradition, but most of which stem from variations in national, ethnic, tribal, and folk cultures. Much as Muslims are Muslims, and even when they are devout Muslims, many social practices and religious beliefs come from the non-Islamic sides of their culture. For example, specifically Egyptian, Pakistani, and Turkish folk cultures influence the understanding of death and commemoration of the dead. So too do contemporary scientific and secular concepts and values. Muslim practice everywhere is a blend of religious beliefs and nonreligious forms of culture. This chapter, then, is not a survey of the subject so much as a sampling of Muslim beliefs and practices. It will emphasize the common religious tradition.

MUSLIM RELIGIOUS BELIEFS

Islamic beliefs have two critical tenets. One is belief in the existence of a single God, Allah, the creator of the universe and of human beings, to whom all persons owe *islam*. *Islam* means submission to God's commands as revealed in the Qur'an, acceptance of his guidance and instruction, submission of one's own self-will to His will, and acceptance for good and bad of the life that he has given. Islamic teaching stresses the virtues of humbleness, patience, endurance, gratitude, and obedience to one's maker. Death is the ultimate test of a Muslim's capacity to accept God's decree with fortitude and trust.

This attitude can lead to fatalism, but it also represents a stoic wisdom that can provide comfort and strength in the face of life's uncertainties, changing fortunes, and inevitable conclusion. Muslim religious culture has always stressed the limitations of human power in the face of fortune and destiny; the changeableness of both good luck and bad; and the need for every person to accept the good things of life with humility and the bad with enduring trust in the meaningfulness of existence. The stoic attitude counsels one not to rejoice too much in good fortune nor to despair in bad times, but to accept the conditions of one's existence with restraint and dignity.

The second central Muslim tenet is that death is not the end of an individual's life but rather a transition into a new phase of existence. In the Muslim view the human being is composed of both spiritual soul and material body. When the body dies, the life-infusing spirit of man (*ruh*) lives on. Muslims believe that all individuals will be resurrected, body and soul together, at the Day of Judgment. Those who have lived a good and believing life will be rewarded with eternal bliss in paradise, and those who have done evil will be condemned to the fire.

The life of the first phase—life in this world—may be decisive for the reward or punishments that the individual experiences in the life to come. While pre-Islamic Arabian and early Muslim cultures had a strong conviction that the length of one's life is fated and unchangeable (a duration called *ajal*, a fixed time), the fate of the human being after death is in the realm of human responsibility. The quality of this life is critical but still secondary, for it is temporary. Life in the next world, however, is eternal— and more important because after death the individual will be integrated into the world of spiritual and heavenly existences where the human soul can find its ultimate meaning. Death can be accepted with solemnity and calm for it is the transition to a truer life.

These views are, in general, similar to Christian views about death, but there are a number of distinctive aspects to the Muslim religious understanding. One is the Muslim concept of the *barzakh,* the isthmus: the transition between life in this world, *al-dunya,* and life in the world to come, *al-akhira.* Between death and the resurrection there is an intermediate phase, the life of the grave. Death and the life of the grave are a fearsome experience. Forty days before the end of a person's life, a leaf bearing the name of the soul falls from the heavenly tree of life and death. The person's fate is fixed. At the moment of death, the angel of death (Izra'il in some accounts) and other angels appear to the dying person. He cannot resist or persuade them to give him more time. The separation of the soul from the body is excruciating, and the dying person suffers intensely. Though the soul rises temporarily to heaven, it returns to the body in the grave.

In the grave the dead person is visited by two angels, Munkar and Nikar, who test the buried person on his faith and question him about his deeds in life. They determine his condition in the grave. Martyrs for Islam go directly to heaven. Good persons may be relieved of the oppressiveness of the grave by the opening of a window to heaven through which refreshing breezes waft and comfort them. Or the investigating angels may consign the person to unspecified torments for an evil life. After punishment the person remains unconscious until the day of resurrection. Comfort or punishment are experienced by both body and soul. The life of the grave thus prefigures the coming Day of Judgment. (Not all Muslim theologians and scholars accept this version in all details. Also many Muslim philosophers, mystics, and Shi'a do not believe in the reunion of body and soul, and do not accept the punishment in the grave.)

The Day of Judgment is more terrifying still. The signs of the hour are described in eloquent and fearsome passages in the Qur'an.

THE DARKENING

In the Name of God, the Merciful, the Compassionate

When the sun shall be darkened,
when the stars shall be thrown down,
when the mountains shall be set moving,
when the pregnant camels shall be neglected,
when the savage beasts shall be mustered,
when the seas shall be set boiling,
when the souls shall be coupled,
when the buried infant shall be asked for what sin she was slain,
when the scrolls shall be unrolled,

> when heaven shall be stripped off,
> when Hell shall be set blazing,
> when Paradise shall be brought nigh,
> then shall a soul know what it has produced.
> (Qur'an, Sura 81:1–14; Arberry 1955, 2:326).

On earth the coming of the end of days is heralded by terrible events—the breakdown of morality and the degradation of communities. Individuals throw off all moral restraints. The coming of the antichrist and of Yajuj and Majuj, Gog and Magog, mark the end of the world. The sun rises in the west announcing the destruction of the cosmic order as well. This is the last moment, the moment of the advent of Jesus and the Mahdi, the messiah.

In the heavenly world an angel blows the first blast of the trumpet announcing the disintegration of the cosmos.

> So, when the Trumpet is blown with a single blast
> and the earth and the mountains are lifted up and
>   crushed with a single blow,
> then, on that day, the Terror shall come to pass,
> and heaven shall be split, for upon that day it
>   shall be very frail,
> and the angels shall stand upon its borders, and
> upon that day eight shall carry above them the
>   Throne of thy Lord.
> On that day you shall be exposed, not one secret
>   of yours concealed.
> Then as for him who is given his book in his right hand,
> he shall say, 'Here, take and read my book! Certainly
> I thought that I should encounter my reckoning.' So he
>   shall be in a pleasing life
>   in a lofty Garden,
>   its clusters nigh to gather.
> 'Eat and drink with wholesome appetite for that you did
>   long ago, in the days gone by.'
> But as for him who is given his book in his left hand,
> he shall say, 'Would that I had not been given my book
> and not known my reckoning! Would it had been the end!
>   My wealth has not availed me,
>   my authority is gone from me.'
> 'Take him, and fetter him, and then roast him in Hell.
> (Qur'an, Sura 69:12–30; Arberry 1955, 2:297–98)

At the second blast all being is extinguished except God (*fana'*), and now the Lord opens the treasure houses of his throne causing the earth to quiver with renewed existence. The third blast of the trumpet announces the resurrection of humankind, body and spirit united for the final judgment. As human beings pour out of their graves, naked and dazzled, they are driven to the concourse of the Last Judgment, a smooth and white plain where they must stand in the blazing heat of the sun, streaming perspiration, waiting three hundred years without food or water. In an atmosphere of blazing terror and barren, comfortless, pure being, terrified souls wait for God's judgment.

The inquisition is crushing. An angel reads each person's deeds from the heavenly book. Good and evil are weighed in the *mizan,* the scales of judgment. Then the souls are driven to the bridge of *sirat.* In some accounts, God has already decided their fate. The saved will find the bridge to be broad, paved, and easily traversed; for the damned it will be thinner than a hair, sharper than a sword, and blacker than night. The souls of the damned will fall into the abyss. Many accounts describe a Pool of the Intercession where the prophet may ask God for His mercy for condemned souls. This is the only moment of relief in a landscape that mirrors the desolation of souls as they go to judgment in solitary terror.

The blessed enter into heaven for an eternal existence of bliss and pleasure. For the blessed, body and soul are comforted by green lands, trees, and rivers; rich furnishings of tents and beds; abundant heavenly food; the company of one's loved ones; the companionship of the virgin houris; and, above all, the vision and contemplation of God.

> So God has guarded them from the evil of
> that day, and has procured them radiancy
> and gladness,
> and recompensed them for their patience
> with a Garden, and silk;
> therein they shall recline upon couches,
> therein they shall see neither sun nor
> bitter cold;
> near them shall be its shades, and its clusters hung
> meekly down,
> and there shall be passed around them vessels of
> silver, and goblets of crystal,
> crystal of silver that they have measured
> very exactly.
> And therein they shall be given to drink a cup whose
> mixture is ginger,

therein a fountain whose name is called Salsabil.
Immortal youths shall go about them;
when thou seest them, thou supposest them
scattered pearls,
when thou seest them then thou seest bliss
and a great kingdom.
Upon them shall be green garments of silk
and brocade; they are adorned with
bracelets of silver, and their Lord shall
give them to drink a pure draught.
'Behold, this is a recompense for you, and
your striving is thanked.'
(Qur'an, Sura 76:11–22; Arberry 1955, 2:315–16)

The torments of hell are not described in the Qur'an. They will last indefinitely but not eternally, for God in his mercy is expected to give respite even to the most evil of sinners.

The position of women is uncertain. They are included in the judgment and the afterlife, but it is not clear whether they too will enjoy conjugal relations. Reflecting a misogyny that became more intense in later eras of Middle Eastern Islamic history, the collected sayings of the prophet commonly hold that most women, lacking reason and self-restraint, will end up in hell.

The traditional view continues to be the vision of Muslims the world over. Contemporary writings on the subject affirm the resurrection of the body and the physical rewards and punishments, often with the proviso that the physical life of the world to come is not like our own and cannot be known or imagined.

THE CEREMONIES OF DYING AND DEATH

This vision shapes the ceremonies surrounding death itself. In many Muslim countries there are two parallel rituals of death: one male, one female.

The male ritual follows the hadith or sayings of the prophet. The devout Muslim, sensing the approach of death, prepares himself for the grave. He performs ablutions as he would before prayer so as to be in a state of ritual purity, washed clean of pollution. He recites the *shahada* or profession of faith; he may lie down facing Mecca. The whole community will gather to comfort the dying man and his family.

The funeral and burial follow as soon after death as possible, preferably within the same day, or if the death occurred at night, the following day. A religious funeral is marked by utmost simplicity. The eyes of the dead person are closed, the body is arranged, the jaws are tied shut, and the body is washed. Special care is taken to clean the orifices and to stuff them with cotton. The washed body is then dressed in its shroud, often three layers of cotton, though sometimes more. The body is placed on a bier and carried to the cemetery, preceded and followed by the male members of the community. The funeral cortege will be joined by passersby, for participating is considered a good deed. The procession may stop en route for prayers or it may go to the mosque. Only men go to the mosque, and they recite the prayers without making the ordinary prostrations. The body is then lowered into a simple grave, without a coffin, and laid on its right side facing Mecca. A stone is placed under the head to hold it in place. In Egypt a simple grave will be deep enough to permit the dead person to sit up for the examination of the angels. The grave is then filled, perhaps to the level of a small mound. A flat stone is placed on the grave. In some regions food will be distributed to the poor according to the means of the family.

The hadith and manuals of advice on burials specify the prayer formulas that accompany each stage of the funeral and burial process. Each gesture in the washing is accompanied by an appropriate prayer. The prayers stress humility and *sabr* (a virtue that combines patience, steadfastness, and self-control), ask for God's forgiveness, and extol His majesty. The recitation of the *shahada* is particularly important and is said both by the dying person and on his behalf after death. The last prayer at the grave is the *talquin*, the instructions to the dead person on how to respond to the questions of the examining angels, Munkar and Nikar.

The burial is typical of Muslim rituals in that actions and words are united. This reflects a Muslim understanding that the union of thoughts in the heart with words and actions brings a person into harmony with himself. The joining of inner intention, verbal thoughts, and ritual gestures brings self-control, wholeness of being, and inner peace.

A death is commemorated at intervals in the subsequent weeks. In Egypt the common pattern is a three-day period of mourning followed by visits to the grave on the first and second Thursdays and on the fortieth day. The fortieth day in many Muslim countries marks the last major commemoration and the end of the period of mourning.

The male rituals strive for self-control, dignity, restraint, and the worship of God in the face of loss and grief. While the men uphold the rationality (*aql*) of human nature, the women express the passionate side. They gather to loudly lament the loss of a loved one, and devastation of a family, the grief of a community. The women, often reinforced by professional female mourners, call out the traditional wailing call, cry in a chanted lament, and recite poetry that expresses their anguish, brooding, and despair. The women forgo self-control and may in their grief tear their clothes, pull their hair, and scratch their faces deeply enough to draw blood. They may dance with abandoned grief, sometimes to the level of hysteria.

Men and women are separated in these ceremonies. In some countries women are not permitted to accompany the funeral to the cemetery; in others they come behind the bier. Where women are permitted to accompany the bier, the men hush them. Visits to the cemeteries and the commemoration of the dead are most commonly female activities.

The women's behavior symbolizes the forces of family, nature, and passion rather than religious devotion and submission to God. While the Islamic discourse and rituals surrounding death and funerals suppress personal feeling and try to reassert the supremacy of loyalty to God over all personal attachments, the women's discourse turns from eschatological beliefs to family bonds. The women's lamentations are a demonstration that death has temporarily overwhelmed self-control and faith in God. Whereas the religious discourse signifies the ultimate human commitment to God, the women's discourse expresses inconsolable loss. All funerals are dramatizations of these conflicting points of view.

Numerous hadith denounce women's behavior as a detraction from God's majesty that may imply that God has committed a wrong action. Recent Islamic revival movements make a point of trying to suppress women's behavior. Wherever the revival movements have become strong, there is increased pressure to suppress the female form of mourning. The stoical religious philosophy competes with deep personal attachments and the feelings they engender.

GRAVEYARDS AND CEMETERIES

Cemeteries are another domain for the unresolved conflict of these two points of view. One point of view calls for the dead to be buried in sand without durable structures or durable markers. The proponents of this view also oppose the construction of tombs, the visitation of graves, and the ceremonies of veneration at the graves of saints and holy men.

Other theologians classified the construction of tombs and visitation of graves as *makruh* (disapproved), rather than *haram* (forbidden).

In fact, from earliest times Muslims have constructed funerary monuments. In Cairo, for example, tombs were built for the holy family of Ali, the prophet's cousin, and the cemetery zone of Cairo acquired the reputation for being blessed land—for communicating into the world *baraka*, the divine power of help and healing. Other pious Muslims, trying to assure themselves a place in the world to come, built their own tombs as well as house-like dwellings, mosques, and schools in the City of the Dead. Endowments were set aside to support the reading of the Qur'an and to provide stipends for teachers, students, and holy men. The flourishing of religious activity brought crowds of visitors to al-Qarafa to commemorate their family dead, pray at venerated tombs, and indulge themselves in pleasant outings in a carnival atmosphere. As people moved into the graveyard buildings, al-Qarafa flourished as a new suburb of Cairo—an inhabited, bustling city of the dead.

In Egypt today, the dead are buried in family tombs, often a square chamber built over excavated ground and capped with a dome. A tomb is called a *dar* (house) and represents an extension of the family's existence to the grave.

Despite the fact that Islam is a jealous religion that tries to differentiate itself from other faiths, and despite its opposition to pre-Islamic cultic practices, pagan festivals, the veneration of saints, and to the status-seeking, vanity, pride, display, and inequality signified by funerary architecture, Muslims the world over take for granted that the dead in some way share the lives of the living. This belief is expressed in their architecture, ceremonies, and festivals.

THE VISITATION OF GRAVES AND THE CULT OF SAINTS

The most important manifestation of this faith is the veneration of saints, those mystics who have perfected their inner being and have achieved a true vision of God. Such holy men commonly become teachers, mediators, and healers in their communities. They often acquire a reputation as workers of miracles, capable, as friends of God, of channeling God's power (*baraka*) into the world of human affairs. This faith in intercession leads to the veneration of saints, their disciples, their descendants, and above all their tombs, which are believed to be repositories of the divine presence. Many Muslims believe that the saints may intercede with God on behalf of the living. To this day throughout the Muslim world, the most common form of worship is the visitation of the graves of saints. By virtue of pilgrimage, prayer, and small gifts, the devout Muslim may ask for the saint's miraculous intercession with God. All over the Muslim world, burial places ranging from small domed commemorative tombs to vast complexes including mosques, schools, and other social facilities mark the graves of the saints. Sufi brotherhoods and lineages grow up around the tombs of saints. It is widely believed that the bodies of saints do not disintegrate, and that they lie intact, present, ready to receive the pleas of Muslims.

THE REALM OF THE SPIRITUAL REALITY

The construction of cemeteries, the placing of grave markers, the construction of tombs and park-like cemeteries, and the visitation of graves are all undertaken based on the premise that the souls of the departed are alive and potentially communicating with the world of the living. The behavior of the living can affect the punishment of the dead; their prayers may ease the way. The dead can communicate with the living, appear to them in dreams and visions, and intercede with them before God. Communication with the dead may also reveal the future, result in miraculous help, and open the way for the living to better understand the world of the spirits and the fate that awaits them.

This sense of connection points to a fundamental Muslim view of the nature of the human being. In the literatures of philosophy, theology, theosophy, and mysticism, the human being is understood as a composite creature—belonging partly to the world of created and corrupt matter and partly to the world of spiritual reality. The body is of this world, but the mind, the rational soul, partakes of spiritual reality and belongs to the world of the divine. The human being partakes of both worlds as a result of the very process of the creation of the universe. All worlds emanate, radiate, from God himself, who by self-contemplation generates the first intellect, the first spiritual being that is both part of and separate from the divine being. Each successive intellect, contemplating itself, radiates another level of spiritual reality down to the tenth, or active intellect. The latter generates templates for shaping matter into concrete objects. It also directly illuminates, through the rational faculty, the mind of human beings. These successive levels of spiritual reality are sometimes described as the celestial spheres, angels, or souls.

The human being partakes of this spiritual reality, but the soul is also embedded in the body, and the task of life is to transcend the physical world and enter wholly into the only and ultimate reality. Transcendence—the rising up of the soul to God—can be achieved by living in accord with God's command, by purifying the heart, and by subordinating the bodily desires and the animal faculties. In this way, human beings liberate their capacity for receiving the active intellect and for having a visionary knowledge of God. The process of self-purification shapes the soul and prepares it for mystical knowledge.

The human imagination is the link between the two universes. The imaginative faculty stands below reason, but it receives impulses both from the senses, the windows on the material world, and from rational intelligence, the window on the spiritual world. Imagination is therefore called a *barzakh*—an isthmus or bridge between the two realities. The imagination makes known to us in this life the existence of angels and spiritual beings and conveys divinely inspired dreams, visions, and revelations.

Thus the survival of the soul after death represents a higher state of being than life itself. The soul at death has been shaped by its experience of the world. It has acquired attributes both good and bad from the way it has lived its time in this world, and it will be rewarded and punished in accord with its worldly experience. Perhaps more important, death, by freeing the spirit, permits it a more true vision of reality, a more pure experience of spiritual being, a more direct participation in the reality of the divine being. Death then advances the journey of the soul toward the truth. Passing through the phases of the grave and of punishment, entering heaven, the soul may advance to see and unite with God.

THE MEANING OF DEATH FOR LIFE IN THIS WORLD

In Islam, life in this world is a small but critical part of a larger human existence. A human life should be conducted accordingly with a sense of proportion. It should be conducted appropriately by fulfilling God's commands, by doing good deeds. A good Muslim should live in a sober, restrained way before the judgment and not be given to excess, heedlessness, or neglect of religious duties. A good Muslim should not only live in the world without renouncing the goods of daily living, but also resist becoming attached to or dependent upon worldly satisfactions. He should live in but not care too much for the life of this world. With detachment, humility, and patient waiting, he makes his way through life to the world beyond.

References

Abu-Lughod, J. 1993. Islam and the gendered discourse of death. *International Journal of Middle East Studies* 25:187–205.

Abu-Zohra, N. 1991. The comparative study of Muslim societies and Islamic rituals. *Majallah al-Tarikhiyah* (Tunis) (Dec.):7–38.

al-Ghazali, Abu Hamid Muhammad. 1989. *The remembrance of death and the afterlife*, trans. T. J. Winter. Cambridge: Islamic Texts Society.

Arberry, A. J. 1955. *The Koran interpreted*. 2 vols. New York: Macmillan.

Chittick, W. C. 1988. Death and the world of imagination: Ibn al-'Arabi's eschatology. *Muslim World* 78:51–82.

Death and death ceremonies. 1972. Karachi: Peermahomed Ebrahim Trust.

Geijbels, M. 1982. *Muslim festivals and ceremonies in Pakistan*. Rawalpindi, Pakistan: Christian Study Centre.

Goodwin, G. 1988. Gardens of the dead in Ottoman times. *Muqarnas* 5:61–69.

Lane, E. W. 1966. *Manners and customs of the modern Egyptians*. New York: Dutton, Everyman's Library.

Lapidus, I. M. 1988. *A history of Islamic societies*. Cambridge, Eng.: Cambridge University Press.

Leister, T. 1990. Between orthodoxy and exegesis: Some aspects of attitudes in the Shari'a toward funerary architecture. *Muqarnas* 7:12–22.

Marcus, A. 1989. *The Middle East on the eve of modernity*. New York: Columbia University Press.

Smith, J. I., and Y. Y. Haddad. 1981. *The Islamic understanding of death and resurrection*. Albany: State University of New York Press.

Williams, C. 1985. The cult of 'Alid saints in the Fatimid monuments of Cairo. Part 2: The mausolea. *Muqarnas* 3:39–60.

Yatim, O. M. 1988. *Batu Aceh: Early Islamic gravestones in peninsular Malaysia*. Kuala Lumpur: Museum Association of Malaysia.

Chapter 18

From This World to the Next:
Notes on Death and Dying in Early America

John Demos

This stop on our multicultural tour of death and dying is marked as "early America"—which for present purposes means the British colonies along the North American coast during the first two-thirds of the eighteenth century. I wish to say, before trying to take you there, how struck I am by the recurrence throughout our "tour" of certain broad themes and tendencies: themes such as the process of preparing for death (or, in some cases, not preparing); the need for personal solidarity when facing death; the apparent permeability of the world of the living and that of the dead. These points you will notice in the early American "stop" as well.

In one respect, I shall take a somewhat different approach from all the other tour guides in that I will present in considerable detail two particular deathbed "scenes." It's true that they are only two, and that both have some distinctive features; nevertheless, when you put them together, you can surely capture the flavor of many such scenes from that same long-ago time and place.

There is one more preliminary comment I wish to make—something that indeed feels almost like a confession. I myself have never attended a scene like the ones I'm about to present from "history." I have never personally witnessed death, or the moments and hours just before death. Clearly, in this respect I'm different from many (especially physicians), but I may not be so different from a lot of more or less "ordinary people" nowadays. If we stopped passersby at random and asked them whether they had personally witnessed episodes of death, I suspect that a good many would prove hardly more experienced in this matter than I. Of one thing I *am* sure: that same lack of experience would have been rare, indeed almost inconceivable, in the early American setting to which I now turn.

The first of my "scenes"—they might also be called "case studies"—is drawn from the 1727 diary of a Massachusetts clergyman, Rev. Ebenezer Parkman (Demos 1991, 188–92). Parkman, if he was like other New England ministers in the eighteenth century, would have had many experiences roughly comparable to the one he describes here. I expect that his language may seem a little unfamiliar, or even off-putting, but I quote it here without alteration—partly for the sake of detail, and partly because of its tonal qualities.

Sometime after sundown Lieutenant Forbush came and requested me to go down to see his wife, who, they thought, was drawing near her end and wanted to see me. I went down and entered the room where she lay. Mr. Thomas Forbush and his wife, Captain Byles and his wife, and Jedediah How were in the room, besides the family. When I entered I said, "Mrs. Forbush, I am sorry to see you so ill. I am come at your desire. Which way can I become the most serviceable to you?" She replied that she was under apprehension of the approach of death and she could not help but be under fears on so great an occasion. Upon which I proceeded to enquire into the grounds of her fears, telling her that I should endeavor to remove them; and to promote the matter the more readily I began to say something concerning true repentance, universal obedience, and the unfeigned love of God—which, finding it in her, might show to her the truth of grace to be wrought in her, which being demonstrated must necessarily make all things bright and clear and comfortable. But this process I managed in such an easy and familiar manner as the following.

1. "I am hoping, Mrs. Forbush, you have freely repented of any sin that you have known yourself guilty of." She answered that she trusted she had, and was heartily willing to repent of all that she had been chargeable with.

2. "You have told me heretofore that you have used your utmost to keep the commands of God universally; but especially now, since you have openly dedicated yourself to God and joined yourself to the communion of the Lord's people and waited upon Christ's table, I conclude you have much ground for satisfaction and comfort. (You should have if you have sincerely and uprightly done your duty.)" To which she said, "It has indeed been a comfort to me, and I am now glad that I have not that work to reproach myself with the commission of, or (in these words) I am glad I haven't that work to do now."

3. "But to find out some further proof of all this and to have some stronger evidence of your love to God and Christ, have you a pure love to the Godly? Do you love the disciples of Christ, those that you think bear the image of God unfeignedly?" She: "I hope really that I do."

The description continues for several pages more, but this excerpt gives the general idea. The forms of questioning and discussion used here were typical of such "scenes" in early America; indeed, they were central to the larger process of preparing for what in the minds of all concerned would follow in the "afterlife."

I should also mention that Mrs. Forbush did not actually die at this point; instead, she recovered quite nicely some days or weeks later and lived (as the saying goes) to a ripe old age. I think there is an important point here. Under the "premodern" conditions of life in early America—and, presumably, in many other premodern contexts as well—one never knew the odds of survival in a particular case. To put the matter in different terms: the relationship between illness, on the one hand, and dying, on the other, was basically unclear. Whenever someone became seriously or substantially ill, there was a possibility that he or she might die; hence the need for the sort of preparation used with Mrs. Forbush. Nowadays, of course, the relationship between illness and death is much more fully understood. A friend may look and feel terrible, but can usually be confident of recovery because we know what the illness is and that one doesn't die from it. At the same time, another friend who looks fine and seems to be getting along well can go to the doctor for a routine "physical" where a problem is discovered and diagnosed as "terminal." So much for outward appearances; but of course these outward appearances were the basis of medicine and of estimates about life-and-death prospects in premodern times.

Now for my second case. This one is presented in a document entitled "The Triumphant Christian: A Record of the Death of Sarah Lippet" (Demos 1991, 192–94). Mrs. Lippet was a Baptist woman who lived in New Jersey in the early and middle decades of the eighteenth century; her death occurred in 1767. The document itself is rather long, but by excerpting from it here and there I hope to convey to you its main thrust.

> The first morning that she was so exceeding ill she said, "my breath is short, and all the time I have I pray that I have patience to bear what the Lord pleases to lay on me. I have had comfort, a little before, and now am willing that His will should be done." At her request one person read the third chapter of Habakkuk; said she, "I will say as Habakkuk did—let it be with one as it will, yet I will serve the Lord." She desired to hear the sufferings of Christ read, whereupon she said, "What great love He had for sinners, to lay down His life for them." . . . At her request she had the second chapter of the first epistle of Peter read, and would often mention these words, "Who Himself bore our sins in His own body on the tree."
>
> The second night of her being so very ill, about one o'clock, it was thought she would have instantly expired. People coming into the room, she said, "They

think I am dying, but I know I am not, and think I shall not die this night. Yet I have no expectation of getting up, and am to go, yea, rather go than stay." About an hour later, she revived and slumbered, then awoke with these words, "It is all calm. I have no terrifying thoughts in my mind, but a great calm." About eight o'clock that morning she said, "Whether it be today or tonight, I am ready and willing; don't mourn for me, but for yourselves and your children." One of her friends came in to take leave of her and asked her how she did. She said, "I am just departing, and have been kept all my lifetime in doubt and fears, but now am delivered." . . . Some she advised to seek for an interest in Christ, and said, "When all things else leave you, that will not; for what advantage will it be to gain the whole world and lose your soul?"

The morning before she died one of her friends came in to see her, to whom she said, "I am just going, I am right free and willing to go. I have no fear on my mind, death is no terror to me. I know if I had my desert I should be in the hottest Hell. I believe in Christ and His blood cleanseth from all sin. This past three months I have been resigning myself up to the Lord day and night, for my death has been revealed." She said to one person that she desired him with her. Then she said, "I have been strengthened to hear and know that your prayer was heard. For I saw the Lord Jesus look down from Heaven and smile on me. I am now on a dying bed and I know not but a dying hour, for I feel one of my eyestrings broke and I don't expect to see the light of another day. It is true I see Jesus, by an eye of faith, look down from Heaven and smile on me."

About two that afternoon she was sensible of a very great alteration in herself, although she continued till past one o'clock that night. One person asked her if she did not long for that hour, to which she said, "I await the Lord's pleasure. It don't seem like dying to me but going on a long journey. I can seem to see how it will be with me when I am in Heaven. I am going to a world of spirits, and death is no terror to me; all tears shall be wiped from their eyes."

That evening before she died she desired one person to pray with her, for she was very sensible that it would be the last time. Said she, "my friends, you must all lie on a dying bed as you see me now, and I have nothing to do but die. Don't mourn for me when I am dead, for I rejoice." After some time she said, "I must bid you all farewell." She said, "how impatient I am, I now long for the hour; come quickly, Lord Jesus." She died very hard and said, "I never asked the Lord for an easy passage, or else I believe I should have had it granted—come quickly, Lord Jesus, and receive my soul." Then she slumbered for a few minutes. When she awoke they thought she would have gone off then. She said, "Don't let me go asleep again, for I want to know when I die." Then one person asked her if her faith was strong yet. "Oh yes, I tell what I see and feel; my breath is short." She bid them ask her when they see her going; "then," said she, "you will know I am not deceived." She then broke out in these words: "I see the lights; Lord

Jesus, receive my soul and body. I commit into thy care, Lord Jesus, my spirit." And so she died with a smile on her lips.

Let me close my chapter with a few additional comments about both these cases, which reflect the broader pattern of death and dying in early America. It is immediately apparent that these are both scenes of death in a crowd, death in a very social context. There are dozens of people present; especially in the case of Mrs. Lippet, folks are coming and going virtually all the time. Sherwin Nuland referred to the "drama of death," with the dying person as the "star." Could we find a better instance of that than the Lippet case? She lay there hour after hour and day after day, literally ordering people about: read this or that passage from the Bible, bring so-and-so to see me, pray with me now, and so forth. In fact, she is not only the "star," but also the scriptwriter and director.

There was a minister present (as noted in a portion of the document I didn't include here). His role with Mrs. Lippet seems not to have been especially prominent, and that was unusual. In this respect, the case of Mrs. Forbush seems more typical; there Rev. Parkman is at least a costar in his own right. Moreover, alongside the minister and the (supposedly) dying person are all those others, the hovering friends and family members. They, too, have their roles—supporting roles—or simply the role of a "chorus" as in a classical tragedy. In all this, the metaphor of theater does seem apposite—and powerful.

I'm struck in Mrs. Lippet's case by the element not simply of acting but of "broadcasting" as well. She describes, she *announces,* each detail of her dying as and when it occurs. "I see the lights"; "I feel one of my eyestrings broke"; "I see Jesus look down from Heaven and smile on me." Every little quiver is thus presented to the obviously breathless members of her audience. But again, they are also something more than an audience. They offer her support, which she clearly wants and needs. And at the same time they are recipients of an offering from her. They stand to benefit from her struggle, her example, her expression of a special sort of insight that comes with the approach of death. Here is a central point about the "social" aspect of such scenes: the element of *transaction* between the dying person and the others who will live on. There is a profound sense of reciprocity: both sides are in a position to gain from the unfolding exchange.

One is also startled to see right up front in the Lippet case something very like joy in the dying person. At least Mrs. Lippet says, more than once, "I rejoice." Clearly, she feels this to be a supreme moment—a literally culminating moment—in her long life, and she means to experience it as fully as possible. If there is a single line among the many she speaks that especially captures her experience, perhaps it is this: "Don't let me go asleep again, for I want to know when I die." This seems astonishing to us; she wants to be conscious at the very moment of death, to feel it happen— and yes, to enjoy it—which, by our own lights (but not by hers), is something of a contradiction.

In other cases, "enjoyment" may have been less evident, but rarely was it absent altogether. In Mrs. Forbush's case, one feels a powerful current of anxiety; she speaks candidly to the minister of her "apprehensions and fears." In addition, there is grief around the prospect of separation (especially in the survivors). There is hope for renewal and reunion in the afterlife. And there is a feeling of intensity, of extreme interest—of high excitement.

This matter of excitement forms a bridge to the final issue I want to mention here: the frame of "cosmology" within which the premodern Americans understood all such events. They lived a kind of bifurcated existence that included the "visible world" and another that was "invisible." An absolutely fundamental boundary divided the two, and a certain amount of regular traffic passed back and forth. Death was a process of personal movement across the boundary; Sarah Lippet likened it to "a long journey." And as it happened, not only would the dying person cross the boundary once and for all, but also those who remained in the "visible world" had a rare chance for a glimpse of the other side. This opportunity, I believe, accounts for the high level of excitement—and explains, too, the "broadcasting" efforts of someone like Sarah Lippet. Here indeed was the deepest and most powerful aspect of these deathbed "transactions": nothing less than the chance to see, to feel—one might even say to touch—the wellsprings of ultimate reality.

Reference

Demos, J. 1991. *Remarkable Providences: Readings on early american history.* Boston: Northeastern University Press.

Chapter 19

Ars Memoriandi: The NAMES Project AIDS Quilt

Peter S. Hawkins

This chapter is for Luis Varela and Scott Lago.

W hen in November 1985 it was announced that the AIDS death toll in San Francisco had reached the one thousand mark, it occurred to gay activist Cleve Jones that, if that many corpses were to litter a field, the public finally would perceive the extent of the loss.[1] As it was, with death kept behind closed doors, it seemed, according to Jones, that "we could all die without anyone really knowing" (Jensen 1988, 3). Wanting to counter this anonymity, Jones asked participants in the annual march held in honor of Harvey Milk to make placards bearing the name of someone they knew who had died of AIDS; these were then hung on the facade of the old Federal Building. The effect was stunning: a wall of memory that, simply by naming names, exposed both private loss and public indifference.

Rather than connecting this wall display with Maya Lin's Vietnam Veterans Memorial—the obvious precursor—Cleve Jones had another association: the sight of the massed placards instantly reminded him of a patchwork quilt handed down within his family and used to comfort those who were ill or housebound. Yet the quilt Jones "saw" was more than the recollection of a private family possession; it was also a public metaphor. At a later time he would suggest its meaning by saying that "quilts represent coziness, humanity, and warmth"; they are "something that is given as a gift, passed down through generations, that speaks of family loyalty" (Ruskin 1988, 12). But surely from the beginning it was not lost on him that quilts have also come to represent America itself. The patchwork quilt is our quintessential folk art, linked to nineteenth-century sewing bees and a nostalgia for a past sense of community. Perhaps the only thing like it in our national mythology is that other needlework of fabric, color, and pattern that Betsy Ross turned into America's most revered symbol—the American flag.[2]

In the patchwork quilt, then, Jones discovered the domestic equivalent for the sign of national unity. It offered a metaphor of *e pluribus unum*, but it was also a brilliant strategy for bringing AIDS not only to public attention but into the mainstream of American myth—for turning what was perceived to be a "gay disease" into a shared national tragedy.[3] Jones made the first panel of what was to become the NAMES Project AIDS Memorial Quilt in February of 1987. In memory of his best friend, he spray painted the boldly stenciled name of Marvin Feldman on a white sheet that measured three feet by six feet, the size of a grave; the only adornment was an abstract design of five stars of David, each one dominated by a pink-red triangle. Jones's panel, at once a tombstone and a quilt patch, served as a model for the improvised handiwork of others, members of a highly organized gay and lesbian community who also felt the need to respond publicly to the epidemic.

The NAMES Project was formally organized on June 21, 1987, and went public only a week later when its first forty panels were displayed in San Francisco's Lesbian and Gay Freedom Day Parade. National coverage came with an Associated Press feature story in August, by which time four hundred panels had been received. By October of 1987, only two months later, the NAMES Project Quilt was displayed on the Mall in Washington, D.C., not far from the Vietnam Veterans Memorial, as part of the National March for Lesbian and Gay Rights: almost two thousand panels, covering a rectangular area the size of two football fields, extended between the Washington Monument and the Capitol (Fig. 19.1). In 1988, there were more than eight thousand panels arranged in a huge polygon just behind the White House on the Ellipse; in 1989, ten thousand were laid out in a square. For the October 1992 display, the official count was slightly over twenty thousand—with an additional sixteen hundred brought to the site for last-minute inclusion. As of October 1, 1995, almost thirty-two thousand panels have been received.

The Quilt's provocative appearance on the Mall gave the project's leadership an opportunity to denounce the country's indifference to the AIDS epidemic and to rally for greater attention to research and support.[4] For others it offered a way to suffer intimate losses in the most public space in America, to leave behind ghetto and closet, to bring mourning from the margin to the center. But apart from any of the political uses to which it has been put—to raise consciousness or money—the Quilt in any of its forms is most profoundly about the naming of names: the sight of them on the myriad panels, the sound of them read aloud. As with the Vietnam monument, the names themselves *are* the memorial. In both cases they are the destination of pilgrimage, the occasion for candlelight vigil and song. They also serve as surrogate graveyards, "consecrated" ground where the living

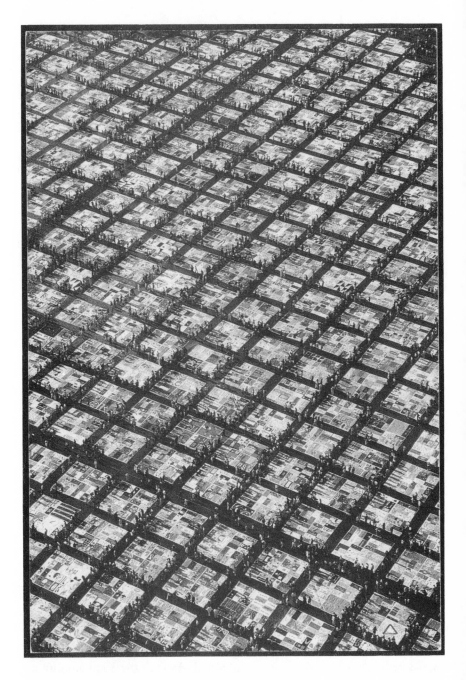

Figure 19.1. NAMES Project AIDS Memorial Quilt. Courtesy The NAMES Project Foundation © 1992. Nita Winter Photography, San Francisco.

can come to pay their respects to the dead—many of whom, their bodies missing in action or their ashes scattered in the wind, have no actual burial site. Indeed, both the Wall and Quilt are commonly treated as places to speak out loud to the dead or to leave behind written messages for them to read—as if the name of the deceased itself provided a medium of communication with another world.[5]

Despite all that the Quilt shares with the Wall, however, its particular naming of names marks a radical innovation in the art of national memory. This is not to deny that Maya Lin's work has been a dramatic departure from the mystique of heroism and triumph that otherwise rules the Mall. Nonetheless, it is precisely on the Mall that the Vietnam Veterans Memorial has its permanent location, at the heart of what passes for our Acropolis or Forum. Nor should we forget that despite its private and quite improvisational beginnings, the Wall's design was the result of national competition, its ongoing maintenance is paid for with public funds, and its roster of names is elegantly incised into granite—a stone that signifies unyielding perseverance in the face of time and change. The memory of *these* dead, to use the unspoken rhetoric of all such memorials, will endure forever.

The Quilt, by contrast, has no official status, no public funding, no fixed location in Washington—indeed, no single place where it can be seen as a whole. Unlike the Wall, which is now complete, the Quilt's response to AIDS keeps growing with the losses from the epidemic. Its increasing size, and the fact that it can barely be contained or even experienced all at once, serve to dramatize a present reality over which we seem to have no control. While the Vietnam war is over, AIDS has only just begun to take its toll. The names that currently comprise the Quilt, just a fraction of the total number of Americans acknowledged to have died from the virus, are but the first casualties to be enrolled.

Given the extraordinary control exerted by Maya Lin over her work from start to finish, it is startling to realize that a memorial on the scale of the NAMES Project Quilt is "authorless," without designer or design. It is true that Jones "invented" the initial three-by-six-foot panel, which he then imagined as one patch taking its place in a larger patchwork.[6] Since then, however, he has had no control over how the Quilt looks, either in its parts or in its larger configurations. Nor has the NAMES Project wielded any authority over the Quilt's appearance, beyond requiring specific dimensions for each panel and that the name of the person to be remembered be specified. Otherwise, design depends entirely on the quilters.

The range of panel designs, as well as the materials used in construction, vary as widely as the makers' skill and sophistication. Shirts and ties, teddy bears, crushed beer cans, merit badges and credit cards, photographs and computer-generated images, leather and lamé, wedding rings, cremation ashes: anything goes. Unlike the paraphernalia of memory that mourners bring each day to the Wall and that each day is taken away, the personal souvenirs incorporated into the Quilt are intrinsic to its formal act of memory—"snapshots of the soul" that no one touches up, censors, or edits.[7]

The same freedom seen in the making of individual panels also characterizes how the Quilt is shown. Aside from the grommeting together of panels in twelve-foot squares for major displays, there is no larger principle of organization at work: no hierarchy, subordination, or ranking; no "metanarrative" that tells a single story or even settles on a particular tone. The Quilt is the ultimate collage, one that is constantly being reformed, reinvented. Its center is wherever you find it: no one tells the viewer where to start, finish, or pay particular attention. Nor does it require of the viewer anything like an "appropriate" response. For despite the enormous grief that inspired and attends it, tackiness and camp also play their irrepressible roles; the carnival always interrupts the wake. For instance, in a small "sampler" display at San Francisco's De Young Museum (August 1–3, 1990) there was a panel made for a Quaker man named Esperando Roseberry that included his wistful last words, "Perhaps now I'll see the Peaceable Kingdom." Next to it, and pointing toward another beatitude altogether, was a memorial to George Kelly, Jr., whose appliquéd T-shirt, stitched onto the panel, even now pulls no punches: "Fuck Art. Let's Dance." Juxtapositions like these, repeated hundreds of times over, prevent any clear or conventional response: the viewer is free to laugh, cry, or do both at once.[8]

This freedom is also reflected in how the name of the deceased appears. In many cases the name is rendered "legally," as on a birth certificate, marriage license, or tombstone. Often, however, the Quilt's names are more private than public, as likely to have been spoken as written down. For every "David R. Thompson" or "Willi Smith" there is a "Patty," a "Clint," a "Fuzzy," or a "Best Daddy in the World." First names or nicknames insist on informality, as if in refusal of the grand occasion or in tribute to a cherished intimacy. But private usage can also conceal rather than reveal—withholding an identity that a surname would give away, protecting a family from its fear of exposure.

That such names appear on fabric rather than being cut into granite is also key. Unlike stone, with its illusion of an eternal witness, cloth fades and frays with time; its fragility, its constant need for mending, tell the real truth about "material" life. Cleve Jones exploited the novelty of a fabric memorial in his remarks at the 1988 Washington display: "Today we have borne in our arms and on our shoulders a new monument to our nation's capital. It is not made of stone or metal and was not raised by engineers. Our monument was sewn of soft fabric and thread, and it was created in homes across America wherever friends and families gathered together to remember their loved ones lost to AIDS" (Jones 1988). In this description, the Quilt becomes a kind of cross, "borne in our arms and on our shoulders." But what really interests Jones is the possibility of something new under the sun, a monument sewn of "soft fabric" at home rather than one erected on the Mall in "stone or metal" by engineers.

What Jones did not say outright is that cloth and thread, as opposed to stone and steel, are traditionally the materials worked by women. And indeed it has been women who, within the private worlds of their own homes and circles, have long used quilting as a way to name names and remember lives. For instance, a woman might make a memory quilt for another person in order to celebrate his or her life. Worked into the design would be bits and pieces of a world: cotton dress material or a silk necktie, cigar bands, dance cards, jewelry, even photographic likenesses. Here the quilt itself becomes a portrait, a fabric reconstruction of another's life that functions almost like a talisman.

If the memory quilt honored a living friend or paid tribute to a prominent member of the community, the mourning quilt served to maintain contact with the dead, to re-member them by sewing together fragments of their lives. These works were usually pieced from the clothing belonging to the deceased, with the design centered on a block whose cross-stitched inscription gives the name, date of death, and often a sorrowful verse. But sometimes the bereaved quilter would make her own clothing the material of memory. This can be seen most strikingly in the work of a turn-of-the-century widow who took her black silk mourning coat, opened it up at the seams, and so covered it with embroidered imagery as to turn the surface of the fabric into a complex of signs—a mass of stitched butterflies, an Easter lily, flags and sailboats, pairs of hearts, a cluster of knives.[9] These symbols, some traditional and others intensely private, express the woman's grief and suggest the complex reality of her husband's life.

Some mourning quilts may very well have been made in anticipation of a loss, as if to forearm against it. This seems to be the rationale behind the 1839 work of Elizabeth Roseberry Mitchell, who created a bedspread that had at its center a representation of the family cemetery. Within its confines appear the coffins of family members already deceased, while at the quilt's borders there are other appliqué coffins representing those still alive. By sleeping under this comforter night after night, Mitchell could perhaps minimize the sting of death by anticipating its coming. More commonly, however, the mourning quilt would serve not as an anticipation of grief but as a response to it. As in the example of the widow's transformed coat, making a quilt might be a major part of the bereavement process itself.

Yet if the NAMES Project Quilt stands in a tradition, it does so on its own new terms. To begin with, it has taken a female art form and opened it up to men, "that ignorant and incapable sex which could not quilt" (Stowe 1982, 789). For centuries, of course, women have made quilts for men to recognize a coming of age, to celebrate an achievement, to mark a death. What the NAMES Project has done, however, is play with gender: men are not only remembered with the Quilt, they are also—together with women— the makers of it. That the male quilters are by and large gay seems at first to confirm a stereotype of effeminacy: while straight men erect public monuments in stone and steel, homosexuals ply needle and thread, do "women's work." Yet by turning the domestic sewing bee into a national effort— and one with strong affinity to the most popular veterans memorial—the NAMES Project in effect makes quilting the work of American "citizens," a large-scale response to public crisis more in keeping with "masculine" monuments than with traditional quiltmaking.

In contrast to most nineteenth-century antecedents, the NAMES Project Quilt emphasizes the sheer specificity by which persons are remembered. A Victorian mourning quilt, for instance, might incorporate clothing of the deceased, be centered on a name and date of death, and stitch together signs, symbols, and texts. But all such details were contained by and subordinated to the quilt itself. Names could be named, but they also disappeared into the form; personal clothing ultimately became fabric once again.

In the AIDS Quilt, however, the three-by-six-foot panel is nothing less than the stage setting of an individual life. The name looms large, sometimes to the exclusion of anything else. Clothing also remains unmistakably clothing, as a name is spelled out in neckties or as a pair of worn Levis suggests not only a wardrobe but a particular body and an entire lifestyle. Photographs and likenesses abound. Some of the panels are reconstructions of human narrative that rely as much on private associations as on any public discourse—life stories that need to be decoded. Moreover, intimacies are everywhere confided to strangers. The panels betray a delight in the telling of tales, revealing in those who have died a taste for leather or for chintz, for motor bikes or drag shows. Secrets are shared with everybody. It is as if the survivors had decided that the greatest gift they could offer the dead would be telling everything, breaking the silence that has surrounded gay life long before the advent of AIDS. Piety now demands that the truth be spoken without embarrassment or circumlocution.

Contrary to the common NAMES Project disclaimer, "politics" is by no means foreign to the AIDS Memorial Quilt. It was born in the gay rights movement and despite both the changing demography of AIDS and the project's desire to reach out to the growing AIDS population of straight intravenous drug users, women, and children, the Quilt continues to be overwhelmingly a memorial to homosexual men. This is not to say, however, that the Quilt is endorsed by the entire gay community. For some activists it is too mild and tearful, too focused on the dead rather than on those still alive or at risk. According to *Village Voice* columnist Michael Musto, for instance, the Quilt should always come with a warning sticker that reads, "DON'T FEEL THAT BY CRYING OVER THIS YOU'VE REALLY DONE SOMETHING FOR AIDS."[10] This uneasiness may arise from the perceived "femininity" of the Quilt, out of a fear that the NAMES Project has organized an androgynous sisterhood rather than keeping faith with a gay brotherhood of sexual rebels and outlaws. *Real* queers don't quilt; they act up. Others, like Douglas Crimp in his influential essay, "Mourning and Militancy," have argued the necessity of grief alongside militancy, granting the AIDS Memorial Quilt a unique role in carrying out "the psychic work of mourning."[11]

In any event, what characterizes the overt political witness of the NAMES Project is the degree to which social or political statements are not only personalized but actually personified. When each panel bespeaks an individual life, it is impossible for even abstract statements to remain abstract. Instead, positions become last wills and testaments; causes are transformed into epitaphs. For Paul Burdett: "The San Diego 50 Hour AIDS Prayer Vigil was His Creation. Please—More Prayers, More Funding." For Billy Denver Donald: "My Anger is, that the government failed to educate us." A panel for Roger Lyon cites the testimony he gave before Congress on 2 August 1983: "I CAME HERE TODAY TO ASK THAT THIS NATION, WITH ALL ITS RESOURCES AND COMPASSION, NOT LET MY EPITAPH READ, 'HE DIED OF RED TAPE.' " The point here is not to weep: rather, panels become platforms, the record of voices raised in a forum where the dead can still have their say.

By and large, however, to make a point is neither the purpose of the Quilt nor the effect of its display. As with the Vietnam Veterans Memorial, it evokes a numbing sense of loss. But whereas the Wall makes its primary impression by force of number, it is the sense of irreplaceable *personal* lives that makes the Quilt unforgettable. The individual parts end up being more than their collective sum.

The poignancy of this personal focus is brilliantly realized in a panel for Jac Wall (Fig. 19.2).[12] Occupying almost the entire space is the life-size silhouette of a man, viewed frontally shin to crown, standing against what

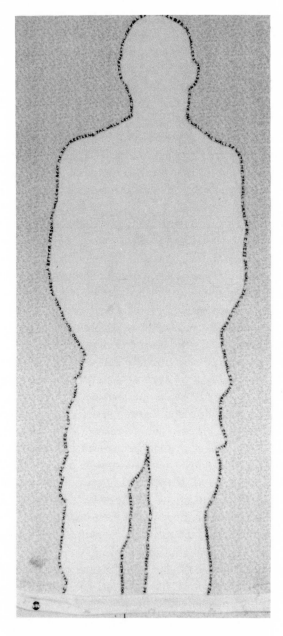

Figure 19.2. *Jac Wall*. Photo: © 1988, Matt Herron/
TAKE STOCK.

appears to be a wallpaper pattern of tiny flowers. The silhouette is cut in reverse, in white rather than black. There is no one to see, no distinctive feature to note, no volume or weight; yet the whiteness of the form makes it radiant, as if light itself were projecting outward, away from the minute detail of the background and moving forward into the viewer's space. The effect is paradoxically to make the represented man both an absence and a presence; in either case, the frame of the panel cannot entirely contain him.

From a distance the form reveals only a generic man. Coming closer, however, one realizes that the silhouette is defined by a text. The dark outline that edges the light, that brings a human shape into recognition, is, in fact, a series of terse statements about a particular person whose identity is conjured up by the continuous repetition of his name. Beginning at the bottom left of the figure and reading up, one traces a description of a life and of a relationship.

> Jac Wall is my lover. Jac Wall had AIDS. Jac Wall died. I love Jac Wall. Jac Wall is a good guy. Jac Wall made me a better person. Jac Wall could beat me in wrestling. Jac Wall loves me. Jac Wall is thoughtful. Jac Wall is great in bed. Jac Wall is intelligent. I love Jac Wall. Jac Wall is with me. Jac Wall turns me on. I miss Jac Wall. Jac Wall is faithful. Jac Wall is a natural Indian. Jac Wall is young at heart. Jac Wall looks good naked. I love Jac Wall. Jac Wall improved my life. Jac Wall is my lover. Jac Wall loves me. I miss Jac Wall. I will be with you soon.

This unfolding line of text enables the survivor to represent the person he lost. Oscillating between past and present tenses, he creates a composite "now" in which the dead man is still powerful, still loving and benevolent. As with the NAMES Project in general, the most private things are said out loud, without concern for convention or decorum ("Jac Wall is great in bed"). But what in fact is said most often is the dead man's name. The reiteration of Jac Wall literally re-members him, brings the shape of his body into view and recalls the features of his life. And so the "I" of the quilter holds on to his lover through his lover's name until the final sentence, with its sudden projection into the future, transforms Jac Wall into you: "I will be with you soon."

The power of this single panel lies first of all in its memorial function. In the face of death it asserts the enduring importance of a particular person, of a loving relationship, of intimate human connection. But taken out of the quilter's private world, the panel becomes evocative of much more. Indeed, placed on the Washington Mall in the company of thousands of other tributes, individual loss becomes national. Such a vision must inevitably disturb the peace, for whenever the Quilt is temporary neighbor to the

Vietnam Veterans Memorial, the White House, and the Capitol, there are certain disturbing connections that become inescapable, links between the war we did not win, the epidemic we cannot cure, and a government that has yet to develop a comprehensive AIDS policy. There are reasons why, when the NAMES Project has come to Washington, presidents have left home or looked the other way.

Nonetheless, the Quilt makes an assault on official oblivion. When on display in Washington it in effect "occupies" the Mall, the traditional site not only of governmental authority but of civil protest against it. At the same time, and if only for a weekend, it creates a place for lesbians and gays to hold hands, kiss in public, feel safe, act like tourists in D.C. Challenging Washington's conspiracy of silence, the Quilt enables the "love that dares not speak its name" to insist outright on public naming, to refuse the very notion of the "unspeakable" and "unmentionable" whether in reference to the fact of AIDS or to homosexual reality.

So too, despite the often sentimental piety that informs so many of the individual panels, the NAMES Project has kept free of the quasi-religious consolations often used in Washington to soften the blows of reality. The Quilt appeals to no "cause" or higher purpose, to nothing that might justify the loss of life or provide some image of transcendence. No flag is ever raised over this Iwo Jima. Instead, merely private identity is held up as monumental; the intimate stretches as far as the eye can see.

Yet despite the warm feelings it evokes, despite its oft-noted "likeability," the NAMES Project Quilt has been taken to task for not covering all the needs of AIDS. Some survivors do not join the project either because of their own alienation from its inclusive myth of a patchwork America or because they respect the real or imagined wishes of the dead. For others it is too sanitized to do justice to gay reality, too male and gay to represent the growing numbers of other inner-city AIDS populations. More irascible critics have found it "whitebread," maudlin, ingratiating, expensive.

But rather than fixing the alleged flaws of the project, it seems wiser to acknowledge the necessary plurality of responses to the epidemic, no one of which can possibly work for all. This plurality is clearly at work with the Vietnam Veterans Memorial. Maya Lin's monument was supplemented by a nearby flag pole and a trio of male figures; it is now augmented still further by a sculpture of three female nurses caring for a wounded soldier. The Vietnam War was too complex an experience to be accommodated in a single way; people evidently needed to say and to see other things. This may also be true of AIDS. Instead of the Quilt simply continuing to expand indefinitely, other gestures may be made representing other ways to live with the epidemic and cherish the lives of those who have died from it.

Even so, it nonetheless seems to me that the NAMES Project Quilt presently provides a unique source of strength and power at a time when so many feel utterly helpless in the face of AIDS. No cure is offered by its acts of memory, nor does the inscription of a name bring anyone back alive. Still, by keeping the names before us, by unfolding them on the ground or speaking them aloud in the air, the Quilt in effect does what it can do for the dead. It insists that all the proper names of love should have the last word. It remembers Michael Mayo, Stephen D'Alessandro, Tim Dlugos, Gregory Cabrera, Velda Bertossi, Bill Sabella, William Boyd, David Rehbein, Daisy Keys, Chuck Hanna, Scott Lago, Paul Monette, John Boswell, Drew Dreeland, and Luis Varela.

Notes

1. A fuller version of this chapter, with more abundant illustration, can be found in Hawkins 1993.
2. Elaine Showalter (1991, 166) recalls that the Bicentennial in 1976 "led to a regendering of the quilt aesthetic in relation to American identity. Every state commissioned a Bicentennial quilt, and many towns and communities made their own album quilts with patches by schoolchildren, senior citizens, women's groups, and ethnic groups. By 1984 a survey indicated that fourteen million Americans had made, bought, sold, or had something to do with a quilt." Jesse Jackson drew on the quilt as metaphor in his speech before the Democratic National Convention in July 1988: he called for the party to make a "quilt of unity," wherein a diverse population, explicitly including gays and lesbians, could discover themselves "bound by a common thread." See "Excerpts from Jackson's Speech: Pushing Party Unity to Find Common Ground," *New York Times*, July 20, 1988, A18.
3. As part of his desire to Americanize AIDS, Jones wanted to dispel the notion that the virus was an invader from overseas: "In the first brochure we wrote, we deliberately used the word 'American' in every paragraph. We wanted to apply a uniquely American concept of this disease that everyone wanted to see as foreign." Cited in Sturken 1992, 79.
4. In a speech delivered October 8, 1988, on the steps of the Lincoln Memorial, Cleve Jones took advantage of this site (near the Vietnam Memorial) to place the Quilt in the context of national tragedy and national response. His point was to challenge governmental apathy in the face of the AIDS crisis: "We stand here tonight in the shadow of monuments, great structures of stone and metal created by the American people to honor our nation's dead and to proclaim the principles of our democracy. Here we remember the soldiers of wars won and lost. Here we trace with our fingers the promises of justice and liberty etched deep by our ancestors in marble and bronze. . . . In the past fifteen months over twenty thousand Americans have been killed by AIDS. Fifteen months from now our new president [George Bush] will deliver his first State of the Union address. And on that day Americans will have lost more sons and daughters to AIDS than we lost fighting in Southeast Asia—those whose names we can read today from a polished stone black wall. . . . History will record that in the last quarter of the twentieth century a new and deadly virus emerged, and that the one nation on earth with the resources, knowledge, and institutions to respond to the new epidemic failed to do so. History will further record that our nation's failure was the result of ignorance, prejudice, greed, and fear. Not in the heartlands of America, but in the Oval Office and the halls of Congress."
5. Jensen (1988) observes that there is a dialogue between the living and the dead set up by both monuments: "[It] reaches an explicit level in 'mediumistic responses' in which the

names are not only addressed, but addressed in a way that presumes the message is received—as though the wall and the quilt are mediums for reaching the dead" (15). The
NAMES Project actively solicits this dialogue by its inclusion of a blank signature panel in
many of its displays—a blank "page" on which visitors may say whatever they want to the
deceased and thereafter have that message on record.

6. The traditional quilt analogue closest to the NAMES Project's patchwork is the sampler
or album quilt, in which blocks of varying design are made separately and then sewn
together. Of particular relevance is the most common type of album in the nineteenth
century, the friendship or autograph quilt, in which individuals contributed standard-sized
swatches (bearing a name and often a message) that were then pieced together into a
"memory" comforter—an ongoing communication between the recipient of the quilt and
absent friends. The wide variety of design found in the NAMES Project panels also recalls the
Victorian "crazy quilt," with its refusal of standardized patterns in favor of the idiosyncratic
and exotic. None of these analogues, however, describes the AIDS Quilt; its enormous size,
ever-changing shape, and heightened individuality of component parts all mark a new quilt
form.

7. Richard D. Mohr (1992) contends that, while the NAMES Project organization does not
dictate standards of "behavior" for the panels, there is nonetheless considerable self-censor-
ship on the part of the panelmakers, with the result that the lives of the deceased are
sanitized. Squeamishness leads the survivors to tell lies of omission: "Aside from scattered
trinkets of leathermen, sex is bleached right out of The Quilt, though sex is what was most
distinctive of most of the dead" (121). It seems to me more accurate to say that the "sex" of the
Quilt is roughly equivalent to that of a New York Lesbian-Gay Pride parade or a New
Orleans Mardi Gras: flamboyant in comparison to the conduct of normal life, but inevitably
constrained by the reality of a public occasion. It may also be that from the perspective of
death, a person's sexual practices may not seem what is most "distinctive" about him or her.

8. It is precisely the power of the Quilt's wild juxtapositions that transformed the initial
skepticism of British AIDS theorist Simon Watney into an appreciation of the NAMES Project
memorial as a "map of America": "To have Liberace alongside Baby Doe, to have Michel
Foucault alongside five gay New York cops. In many ways it's a more accurate map of
America than any other I've ever seen." (Quoted in Seabrook 1990, 111). On the place of
humor as "a form of gay soul," see Rudnick 1993, A21.

9. The widow's mourning coat quilt, now in the collection of Julie Silber, is pictured in
McMorris 1984, 86–87.

10. Musto 1988, cited by Bellm 1989, 35. Cf. Abbott 1988, cited by Sturken 1992, 91: "One
reason the quilt was so readily embraced by the media is because it can also be read as a
memorial to a dying subculture (i.e., 'We didn't like you fags and junkies when you were
wild, kinky, and having fun. We didn't like you when you were angry, marching and demanding rights. But now that you're dying and have joined "nicely" like "a family sewing circle"
we'll accept you')."

11. See Crimp 1989, 7: "Of our communal mourning, perhaps only the NAMES Project
quilt displays something of the psychic work of mourning, insofar as each individual panel
symbolizes—through its incorporation of mementos associated with the lost object—the
activity of hypercathecting and detaching the hopes and memories associated with the loved
one." Crimp concludes his essay: "The fact that our militancy may be a means of dangerous
denial in no way suggests that activism is unwarranted. There is no question but that we
must fight the unspeakable violence we incur from the society in which we find ourselves.
But if we understand that violence is able to reap its horrible rewards through the very
psychic mechanisms that make us part of this society, then we may also be able to recognize—along with our rage—our terror, our guilt, and our profound sadness. Militancy, of
course, then, but mourning too: mourning *and* militancy" (18).

12. I am indebted to Mohr's brief but sensitive reading of this particular panel (1992, 126,
128); Sturken (1992, 81) also notes it.

References

Abbott, S. 1988. Meaning adrift: The NAMES Project Quilt suggests a patchwork of problem and possibilities. *San Francisco Sentinel,* 14 October.

Bellm, D. 1989. And sew it goes. *Mother Jones,* January.

Crimp, D. 1989. Mourning and militancy. *October* 51 (winter).

Hawkins, P. 1993. Naming names: The art of memory and the NAMES Project AIDS Quilt. *Critical Inquiry* 19 (summer): 752–79.

Jensen, M. D. 1988. Making contact: The NAMES Project in comparison to the Vietnam Memorial. Paper presented to the Speech Communication Association, New Orleans, November.

Jones, C. 1988. Address given at the Lincoln Memorial, 8 October. Unpublished material distributed by the NAMES Project.

McMorris, P. 1984. *Crazy quilts.* New York: Dutton.

Mohr, R. D. 1992. *Gay ideas: Outing and other controversies.* Boston: Beacon.

Musto, M. 1988. La dolce Musto. *Village Voice,* 25 October.

Rudnick, P. 1993. Laughing at AIDS. *New York Times,* 23 January, A21.

Ruskin, C. 1988. *The Quilt: Stories from the NAMES Project.* New York: Pocket Books.

Seabrook, J. 1990. The AIDS philosopher. *Vanity Fair,* December.

Showalter, E. 1991. *Sister's choice: Tradition and change in American women's writing.* Oxford: Oxford University Press.

Stowe, H. B. 1982. *Selections.* Ed. Kathryn Kish Sklar. New York: Literary Classics of the United States, dist. by Viking Press.

Sturken, M. 1992. Conversations with the dead: Bearing witness in the AIDS Memorial Quilt. *Socialist Review* 92 (April–June).

Chapter 20

Bearing the Spirit Home

Frederick J. Streets

Each of us brings to the beginning of our professional practice certain assumptions and a level of naiveté. I did not expect the extent to which I had to deal with the dead and those who were dying when I entered the parish ministry. I have since witnessed the deaths of many people and provided pastoral care to their families during my twenty years of pastoral work in an urban environment. The range of my experiences includes some of the best examples of persons dying a "good death." I have also seen some of the worst circumstances in which people die. Here I wish to share some observations about the meaning of the art of dying with the aid of both medical science and religion.

Death is a common denominator for both physician and patient, therapist and client, clergy and congregant. We are confronted as professional helpers with our own feelings, attitudes, and fears about dying when assisting others with their own dying. This causes us to reflect on the meaning dying and death have for our philosophies about life and our healing art. The limitations of our knowledge and skills are brought sharply into focus when we are faced with the inevitable deaths of those for whom we are caring. We will repeat this experience and revisit our questions about life and the value of our profession many times throughout our careers. This means that we must learn to cope with the emotional demands that caring for the dying places upon us and deal with the questions that dying and death raise for us in a manner that fosters our ability to be effective practitioners and to live our own lives well. This is why it is imperative that we as physicians and clergy attend to our own emotional and spiritual needs, however we define them.

It has been stated in this volume that a "good death" has some of the following characteristics: (1) one does not die alone, (2) one dies in relative personal and environmental comfort, (3) one has an opportunity to say good-bye, and (4) dying is enhanced by a "good life"—that is, dying and death are a part of one's entire life.

The medical profession can assist persons who are dying to do so in relative comfort with the use of medication and technology if these means are acceptable to the patient and comply with medical and hospital standards. The opportunity for the dying person to say good-bye to loved ones and friends and to express his or her feelings about dying requires the collaborative support of the medical staff and hospital, as well as the patient's family, and others who are important to the patient. A dying person's religious beliefs, religious practices, and community of faith are important elements in helping him or her to die well.

THE ROLE OF RELIGION IN THE ART OF DYING

A literature review of medicine, social work, psychology, nursing, psychiatry, and pastoral theology reveals that over the past twenty years these disciplines have been reappraising the important roles that religion and spirituality play in the lives of people served by these professions. Space does not allow a discussion of the meaning of these terms, their role in healing, or the sense of purpose they bring to people's lives. But it is important to remember that religious beliefs, religious practices, and notions of spirituality are culturally defined and experienced. They influence the ways in which people understand and live their lives and how they cope with death and dying. One need not be confessional in any religious sense in order to appreciate the value that religion holds for others.

Religious faith helps those who are dying to suffer and die with dignity, grace, and hope. Religion provides at least four things for the dying person. First, it gives a meaning to dying and death that encourages the integration of the experience into the person's larger life. Second, it provides the person with a "healthy" way of coping with dying and death through the use of rituals, prayers, and so forth. Third, it facilitates the transition from life into death and beyond according to the dying person's beliefs. And fourth, religion helps those who are left behind to integrate the suffering, dying, and death of their beloved into the wholeness of their own lives.

Dying is a social act for many people who are religious. The art of dying encompasses the idea that the dying will have their family, friends, and religious community watch and wait with them until death occurs. The vigil may include praying, singing, reading from sacred texts, and periods of silent meditation. This religiously social dimension of the art of dying is crucial for many African-American Christians. They and other Christians see suffering and death as something to be endured and overcome by having faith in Jesus Christ. The identification with Jesus Christ is central to Christians. The importance of this identification historically for the African-American Christian community is captured by Howard Thurman's discussion of the meaning of some Negro spirituals: "The suffering of Jesus on the cross was something more. He suffered, He died, but not alone—they were with Him. They knew what He suffered; it was a cry of the heart that found a response and an echo in their own woes. They entered into the fellowship of His suffering. There was something universal in His suffering, something that reached through all levels of society and encompassed in its sweep the entire human race" (1975, 26). The history and theology of the Christian identity of African-Americans cannot be adequately treated here. It is sufficient to say that they and other Christians believe that at the time of death the soul is separated from the body and returned to God and that the contradictions of life represented most dramatically in death are not ultimate. Death belongs to life. Life and death belong to God.

Wakes and funerals play a vital role in helping the family and friends of the deceased and their community deal with death. The art of dying and death is reviewed, remembered, and learned in subtle ways at the funeral as people gather and participate in the rituals that organize and give meaning to death. Funeral home directors and their staff often play a much larger role in helping families cope with their loss than we realize. In many instances it is they and not the clergy, institutions of religion, or other helpers that assist the family with the dying or with the deceased member and help family members manage and understand their pain and loss. I believe we could better meet the spiritual needs of some of our patients by talking with funeral directors about their experiences working with such families.

The expansive role of the funeral home staff and of the cultural, ethnic, regional, and religious aspects of funerals cannot be further nuanced here, but three of the many important things about funerals in general can be briefly noted. First, funerals socialize the pain of dying and the grief of death for the living. It is an experience shared by the family, extended family, and community of the deceased. During a funeral the meaning of life, suffering, and death is reviewed on some level by everyone involved. Second, funerals educate those present about the meaning of life and death. A theological interpretation and understanding of death and eternal life enable believers to cope with the loss, to "let go" of their loved one, and to go on living by grounding their religious sense of self and hope. Third, funerals help us to understand further the uniqueness and importance we held for the one who has died.

All funerals are also about our own life and death. How we grieve and cope with loss throughout life is reflected in and influenced by the way we bury our dead. We bring these moods and behaviors with us into the hospital room either as patient or helper.

When we attend funerals we are paying our respects and acknowledging our relationship to the deceased. It is also an opportunity to learn something more about how we as human beings grieve. Physicians and other helpers can gain insight about how we as humans grieve by attending the funerals of some of their patients and by reflecting on their other funeral experiences. All dying, deaths, and funerals have theological implications in the sense that they raise for all of us questions about "the author and finisher of life."

A new partnership between health care providers and the clergy is needed to facilitate an understanding of and foster an appreciation for the religious and spiritual sensitivities of patients. The religious or spiritual representative of dying patients is an important resource for a hospital to consult regarding their care. This approach to patient care is not in any way a hospital's attempt to promote religious values. It is, however, a recognition that this aspect of people's lives cannot be neglected if we want to see patients as whole persons and to learn more about the larger human experience.

W. H. Auden, in his "For the Time Being," states, "Life is the destiny you are bound to refuse until you have consented to die." The art of living for some people means for them by living they embraced dying. We come to know something about who they were—how they "consented" to live and what they believed—by the way they "consented to die." Their religious beliefs and spiritual practices express a part of who they are. Further, when they are dying we learn something about the rich and varied forms of the good death and its religious components. We derive meaning not only by working and loving, but also from the art of dying. We learn about ourselves through the life and death of others.

References

Boyd-Franklin, N. 1989. *Black families in therapy: A multisystems approach.* New York: Guilford Press.
Burton, L. A., ed. 1992. *Religion and the family: When God helps.* New York: Haworth Pastoral Press.
Fleischman, P. R. 1993. *Spiritual aspects of psychiatric practice.* Cleveland, S.C.: Bonne Chance Press.
Lowenberg, F. M. 1988. *Religion and social work practice in contemporary American society.* New York: Columbia University Press.
Thurman, H. 1975. *"Deep River" and the Negro spiritual speaks of life and death.* Richmond, Ind.: Friends United Press.

Chapter 21

Witnessing Death versus Framing Death

William B. McCullough

I find much less unhappiness in the chapters of this book by clergy and philosophers than in those by physicians. The medical approach to complex problems relating to death focuses on obstacles and real-life situations. Some situations, familiar to many physicians, represent tragedies of life to which there are no simple answers—or to which all the answers seem to be wrong. Often discussions physicians have relating to the unfairness of death seem to produce a mood almost of anger; anger that the dying are sometimes given answers that seem to be not precisely correct. Discussions by spokespersons of various religious approaches to "framing death" are more peaceful. I do not believe that this difference is a sign that the medical profession is more contentious than the religious has been—a cursory glance at current world conflicts indicates that this is not so. Rather I think it is explained in the difference between "witnessing" and participating, and reflecting and framing. I like the title "framing death" because it is indicative of what religions attempt to do. The physician today more often confronts death in its raw form, as it is happening or about to happen. The religious "framing" of death has the advantage of perspective, distance, and time.

First, however, a few comments about common themes. The distilling of religious thought into basic common denominators tends to be neither accurate nor successful in finding a single, unifying thread. It is the uniqueness and the weltanschauung of each religion that allow it to maintain its consistency. Having said that, there are some interesting themes. Both the Chinese story told in this volume by Valerie Hansen and the puritan account by John Demos have a glimpse beyond the curtain of death into the afterlife. The Chinese man whose topknot was displaced upon his return from death was able to tell his friends and relatives about what he had seen and experienced in the world beyond. And the relatives and friends who gathered around Sarah Lippet at the time of her eighteenth-century death were able to hear her description of the hereafter.

Further, many people want to know they are dying and they want to participate in the death process. In Hinduism, a person "attains his death." In the Judaistic approach to death, it is "a conscious act of giving oneself away." Christianity indicates that a person should be aware of his condition. Both the Chinese and the puritan stories involve awareness of impending passage into the world beyond death, and in fact a decision to "pass on."

A CHANGE IN ATTITUDE

Medicine in the mid-twentieth century has had difficulty dealing with just this aspect of death. Those of us who were in the medical field just twenty-five or thirty years ago remember the discussions about whether a patient who has a terminal cancer should be told! In general, the accepted wisdom of the 1940s was that a patient should not be told of the severity of his or her illness, lest it be depressing and destroy hope. Even the president of the United States, engaged in World War II, was "deliberately not told what his diagnosis was," nor did he ask, when evaluated just months before his death (Goodwin 1994, 496). Amazingly, this secretive approach has essentially disappeared in America today. We assume that patients have the right to know. Patients are encouraged to be treated in "cancer centers" and to participate in cancer awareness groups. Such overt and honest names and titles reflect a great shift in American attitudes about "the patient's right to know."

A group of studies in Los Angeles from 1965 (Feifel 1965) showed that 69 to 90 percent of physicians at that time were not in favor of telling the dying patient that he or she was dying. At the same time, 77 to 89 percent of patients said they wanted to know. Much of the medical community has moved toward openness and a belief that the patient's illness and prognosis (to the degree that medicine can predict it) is the property not of the physician, but of the patient.

MAINTENANCE OF LIFE

These new attitudes about communicating with the dying must now shape a recognition of when to stop with our technology. We have the mechanical capacity to prolong one's heartbeat and respiration long beyond reason, but we often lack the reason to know when to stop. The distinction between prolonging life and prolonging meaningful life is a difficult one. Now that we have mostly passed the barrier of informing patients about their condition, we need to wrestle with when to stop the maintenance of bodily function in the name of maintaining life. A poll at a

1993 meeting of the Association of Academic Surgeons asked physicians whether they felt that in an intensive care unit they should *exhaust all possible means* to keep patients alive. Fifty percent responded in the affirmative. Thus there is still a great need for more "framing of death" in modern medical thought. As our technology continues its rapid advance, the obligation to say to the patient or family that it is time to withdraw our technological pursuit of the maintenance of life will fall increasingly to physicians. Preparing new physicians for this task will be a new undertaking for medical education.

This book illustrates that many within the profession are ready to change the framework in which we deal with death in the 1990s.

A curious thing about late-twentieth-century medicine is that the dead and dying are brought to us who participate in and run the medical establishment. It is said that 80 percent of Americans die in the hospital. This is not, however, the best place to bring the dying. Doctors (especially surgeons) and nurses frequently see death as failure. Our job is to prevent death. When we are unsuccessful, as often occurs, it is very difficult to step out of the role of preventer and into the role of comforter.

In fact most physicians and many nurses have no training whatsoever to deal with death. The dying are often brought to us in the hope that we can do something to change the course of their dying or so that we will "pronounce" them dead. The late-twentieth-century physician thus by default replaces the priest in our increasingly secular society. The art of dying at home surrounded by one's family, friends, and loved ones is rare in late-twentieth-century America. The hospice movement is unique in its invaluable efforts to bring the art of dying to a relaxed and sensitive institutional setting.

There is a basic dichotomy between medicine and religion when it comes to framing death. Medicine is science, although it is in so many ways an inexact science. But the curtain of consciousness that cloaks our awareness of life after death has not and cannot be lifted by science. The religious and scientific ways of knowing are at their base divergent. They are entirely different epistemologies. This is not to say that belief and science do not meet. In fact they come together because they are both a part of the men and women who practice medicine. It is here that medicine and religion work to make a complete physician who is knowledgeable, yet compassionate.

MEASUREMENT AND COMPASSION

Medicine as science is engaged in description, observation, measurement, and categorizing. One can turn to scientific medicine to describe death but not to "frame it."

Religious thought and much secular thought about death turn to poetry for their expression. This is a world where science cannot come, although the scientist can be a part of it. But to speak about the ineffable is to talk in a world where one cannot measure. That world is related to what is called faith or belief: it cannot be quantified. A death is the intersection where measured science meets faith and fear; for none of us can be present at a death without a faint shudder.

Each religion, in its own way, deals with facing and overcoming the fear of death. Why we fear death is unclear. But it is clear that the threat or fear of death is believed to cause the greatest human anxiety. Probably the fear of death is related to a concern that it is an end where the lights go out, where the train enters the dark tunnel and then . . . stops. Perhaps it is, as described by a colleague (Nuland 1994, 10), "permanent unconsciousness in which there is neither void nor vacuum, in which there is simply nothing." Reinhold Niebuhr, one of America's leading twentieth-century theologians, described this possibility as "finis, when that which exists ceases to be" (1953, 287).

This is to Niebuhr in contradistinction to another word for the end—telos—which he describes as the purpose and goal of man's life and work. The end as both finis and telos represents a tension between time and eternity.

After his 1994 interview with Aleksandr Solzhenitsyn, David Remnick described telos as lived by the Russian novelist: "I mentioned to Solzhenitsyn that I remembered his speech in Liechtenstein when he said that modern man, by putting himself at the center of the world, fears death because death thus becomes the end of all things—and I asked him if he feared dying now that he was seventy-five. 'Absolutely not,' he said, his face lighting up with pleasure. 'It will just be a peaceful transition. As a Christian, I believe that there is a life after death, and so I understand that this is not the end of life. The soul has a continuation, the soul lives on. Death is only a stage, some would even say a liberation. In any case, I have no fear of death.'"

Religions all seek to frame life and death together. Life is to be lived with an awareness that it has an end, that it has a finis and a telos. It was Spinoza who used the term *sub specie aeternitatis*—under the view of eternity.

Ars moriendi is, in the end, *ars vivendi*.

References

Feifel, H. 1965. The functions of attitudes towards death. In *Death and Dying: Attitudes of patient and doctor*. New York: Group for the Advancement of Psychiatry.

Goodwin, D. K. 1994. *No ordinary time*. New York: Simon and Schuster.

Niebuhr, R. 1953. *The nature and destiny of man*. New York: Scribner's.

Nuland, S. B. 1994. *How we die: Reflections on life's final chapter*. New York: Knopf.

Remnick, D. 1994. The exile returns. *New Yorker*, 14 February.

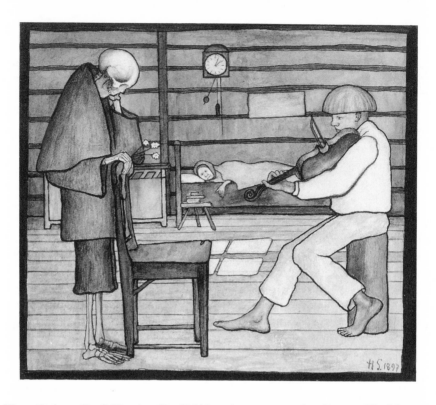

Hugo Simberg, *Death Listening (Der Tod hört zu)*, 1897, watercolor. Courtesy The Museum of Finnish Art Ateneum, Helsinki, Central Art Archives.

Chapter 22

Conclusion: Retrospect and Prospect

William J. Bouwsma

I am not a physician but a European cultural historian. For present purposes I might also describe myself as a kind of general practitioner in an occupation swarming with specialists. I shall try here to combine my resources as a historian with the reactions of a reasonably attentive lay reader of what has been said in this book. I hope that the result will be an adding up of the kind usually expected at the end of a volume.

DEATH AS A PROBLEM FOR MEDICAL PROFESSIONALS

When I accepted the invitation to contribute to this book, its focus—reintroducing doctors and nurses to death—seemed to me, a layman, more than a little odd. Who, after all, should be better acquainted with death than doctors and nurses? But what I have learned here is that although nurses know death very well, as do some doctors—notably those contributing to this book—many doctors, particularly specialists, are troubled by death almost to the point of denial. I am now fully convinced of this after having read Sherwin Nuland's book and having consulted friends in the medical profession. So I have come to understand, at least as far as an outsider can, why the relation of the medical professions to death has become problematic. Death represents a *loss* to those who, through modern technology, have been increasingly used to *winning,* and who might therefore feel tempted to exclude death as far as possible from consciousness. Further, as has been suggested here, there is some evidence that medicine tends to attract people who are themselves unusually anxious about death.

But it also seems to me that this may be only part of the explanation, and here I may be a bit kinder to doctors and nurses than some of the other contributors to this volume. For medical professionals are now called on to perform tasks that previously were assumed by another profession, and especially by the larger, nonprofessional human community. In traditional representations of deathbeds, as has been pointed out here, the dying are surrounded by families, friends, and clergy, constituting a close and supportive community—rather than by medical professionals and machines. This larger community, in our increasingly mobile and atomized society, has now in many cases disappeared. But the need for it remains, though this need can hardly be satisfied by professionals trained to deal with death simply as a medical event terminating the life of an individual.

For death, as a thoughtful physician has recently remarked, has traditionally been far more than this; and it remains, as he wrote, "a momentous occurrence with an impact on the entire group [to which the dying person belongs], which solemnizes it with rituals and public ceremonies. An individual death [in this context] is never trivial since it splits open the treasury of myths and symbols of the community" (Gonzalez-Crussi 1994, 168). For many of us this is still the case even if subliminally. Death requires, from those assisting it, a wisdom, a capacity for reassurance and comfort, an intimate acquaintance with the dying, a priestly role, if you please, which in the absence of priests doctors are now called on to perform and which had never been expected of them in the past. No wonder they feel uncomfortable.

On the other hand, although this problem is still serious, things may already be changing. This book is itself suggestive of changing attitudes among professionals. I will also add another bit of evidence. Having confided to one of my medical friends that I would be attending the conference that launched this book, I was immediately invited to join a Berkeley discussion group, of which I had been unaware. The group, composed mostly of health care professionals, had been formed to discuss precisely the concerns of this conference. It calls itself the Life and Death Potluck Supper Group, and it is very serious. Daniel Callahan, whose recent book *The Troubled Dream of Life: Living with Mortality* has been referred to in this book more than once, met with us some months ago.

DEATH AS TABOO

Death for the laity seems to me a rather different matter. It is indisputable that death was for them a major problem a generation or two ago, as Philippe Ariès and others have demonstrated. It had virtually replaced sex as the major taboo of our culture; it was almost unmentionable and as little thought about as possible. But there is some evidence that for the laity a major change is under way. Ariès himself noted this in the concluding pages of his massive work, which also has been referred to several times in this book. "Phenomena that had been forgotten," he wrote, "have suddenly become known and discussed, the subjects of sociological [and, I would add, historical] investigations, television programs, medical and legal debates. Shown the door by society, death is coming back in through the window, and it is returning just as quickly as it disappeared" (1981, 560).

This was written in 1977; the tendency it describes has since been rapidly accelerating. My own cursory survey of recent literature on the subject of death, most of it written for lay people, surprised me. I have already referred to Callahan's book; and members of the Yale medical faculty have contributed notably to this literature, most recently with Sherwin Nuland's best-selling *How We Die* and Richard Selzer's *Raising the Dead*. Both, along with Frank Gonzalez-Crussi's *Day of the Dead and Other Mortal Reflections*, a chapter of which also appeared in the *New Yorker*, were recent selections of one of the most respected general book clubs. This is of special interest, I think: booksellers know what sells.

Nor is this all. Many books have appeared recently by authors who are not medical professionals. Among them I have noted Fred Feldman's *Conversations with the Reaper*, a work of analytical philosophy; the British sociologist Zygmunt Bauman's deeply reflective *Mortality and Immortality and Other Life Strategies;* and a collection of essays on *Death and Representation*, which reflects the interest the subject holds for critical theorists in a variety of disciplines. I would add that among the doctoral students with whom I am presently working is a very perceptive young woman who is writing about Shakespeare's staging of death, which is interestingly gender specific: men and women in Shakespeare, it turns out, tend to meet quite different kinds of deaths.

DEATH IN HISTORICAL SCHOLARSHIP

To turn to my own discipline, there is now also a large group of studies, going back for more than thirty years, by historians of many countries (Ariès is the best known of these) including Alberto Tenenti, Gaby and Michel Vovelle, John McManners, David Stannard, and a group of historians closer to my own interests whose work has been collected under the title *Life and Death in Renaissance Florence*. This is enough to illustrate my point. Much of this work reflects the popularity of a new kind of social history—history "from below" as it is sometimes described—which has found past practices and attitudes toward death, along with sexual behavior, of particular interest.

There is growing attention, too, to collateral subjects such as aging, the result perhaps of the aging of our own population. So we now have Thomas Cole's excellent *History of Aging in America;* Wayne Booth's anthology, with personal reflections, entitled *The Art of Growing Older: Writers on Living and Aging*—much of which, in various ways, is about death; and, most recently,

The Oxford Book of Aging: Reflections on the Journey of Life, an anthology edited by Thomas R. Cole and Mary G. Winkler. There has also been an exhibition entitled "Portraits of Aging" at the National Humanities Center in North Carolina, and two recent colloquia on aging in America and Europe at my own university. So it would seem that these subjects long denied are rapidly recovering a major place in the contemporary consciousness.

We still, of course, have some distance to go. Funerals continue to take place in a "home" of a kind in which nobody could possibly feel at home, and death is referred to by euphemisms and pet names of the kind attached to other sacred objects such as the deity, the devil, and the male and female genitalia. Perhaps this indirection is useful, possibly to a degree even necessary. I suspect that human beings will never be able to feel entirely comfortable about death, their own or that of others. Nor, I suspect, would we have it otherwise. Death, it has often been observed, gives life its significance.

ANXIETY ABOUT DEATH

But the massive anxiety that has surrounded death at least until recently is another matter because it seems to be historically and culturally specific. Ariès located its origins in the later Middle Ages and the Renaissance, that conventional beginning of the modern age. This period, he believed, saw a crucial shift from the relative acceptance of death in traditional culture to a preoccupation with it in the modern world. Ariès seems to me rather vague about this chronology and about the causes of the changing attitude toward death. But—if I read him correctly—he believed that a kind of collective terror about death and dying gradually became so intolerable that thoughts of death had eventually to be generally repressed and denied. I think he is partly right about this, but that—by his own evidence—people during the eighteenth and nineteenth centuries were a good deal more comfortable with death than in the centuries both before and after.

Nevertheless, I want here to look more closely at the preoccupation with death in the age of the Renaissance, partly because it is that part of the Western past that I know best, but also because it illustrates a point that seems to me crucial in thinking about death. This is that anxiety in general, and anxiety about death in particular, are largely functions of *culture*. This is important for our thinking about how to ameliorate it.

It is now common to distinguish between *anxiety* and *fear*. Fear attaches itself to, results from, our awareness of a concrete and particular danger: fear of robbery, of an automobile accident, of financial loss. Precautions can be taken to reduce or even eliminate such dangers. But anxiety is quite different. It has no such specific focus. It is a result of our awareness of time, and therefore of the unknown that lurks, for us all, in the future. It is a diffuse dread of the unknowable, of what might, of what *will,* happen in the future. Anxiety may attach itself to various threats that we imagine lie in wait for us. But ultimately what lies ahead for us all is death. This is why all anxiety is ultimately about death, which cuts us off from everything known and familiar. Death is the final uncertainty.[1]

Anxiety can, of course, be repressed. It can also be controlled, up to a point, by culture. Cultures, with their rules and regulations, their rituals and taboos, their distinctions and boundaries, can make us feel relatively safe. They provide an orientation without which we would dissolve in a mass of anxieties. And the Renaissance was a period in which a traditional culture that had enabled Europeans to feel relatively at home in the universe, even to a degree in the face of death, was disintegrating. This is the negative side of the great flowering of high culture that we associate with the period; the Renaissance liberated Europeans from the cultural constraints that had kept the dread of death under control.

Before the Renaissance, a traditional culture rooted in antiquity had made the cosmos friendly by picturing it as at once finite, orderly, and unchanging. The various celestial bodies, all divinely controlled from above and ranked in hierarchy, circled the earth, which was man's home in this life. Death, in this conception, was an ascent from a troubled earthly to a paradisaical heavenly home, from one place to another within a fully intelligible universe. In the traditional conception, society too constituted a fixed and hierarchical system in which everybody had a definite place. And the human personality was similarly perceived as a hierarchy of faculties with reason, more or less identified with the soul, in control. God in the universe, king or pope in society, reason in the person: all were more or less reliable sources of order and stability.

But from the fourteenth century on, this neat, orderly, security-making set of conceptions was under attack from various directions. I can't here go very far into why this occurred. Underlying the change, however, was a vast increase in social and geographical mobility that reached a climax with the European penetration of Asia and the discovery of exotic new worlds and peoples utterly different in their ways of life and thought from those of Europe, which had been thought universal. This coincided with the disorientation occasioned by the new cosmology of Copernicus and Galileo and a growing awareness that the universe was infinite. In an infinite universe nothing can be thought of as having, in any absolute sense, its place.

I don't wish to exaggerate. The disorientation that resulted operated very slowly. Nor was it ever total; it is still at work in the skeptical and relativistic impulses at work in our own time, which are still a source of anxiety. In many respects the seventeenth, the eighteenth, and even the nineteenth centuries were more stable and less anxious than those that immediately preceded and followed. New sources of order and stability were discovered, notably in the comforting certainties supposedly provided by science and reason. And there are still residues of the old culture among us, as in the notions of heaven as "up there" and of the fixity of biological species that some of our contemporaries can still read into the biblical story of the creation.

Meanwhile the collapse of the traditional culture with its comforting boundaries and its picturable future in heaven made death seem far more dreadful, the focus of terrible imaginings. The *ars moriendi,* so vividly described and illustrated by Arthur Imhof, was largely a product of this period and testifies to its preoccupation with death. This was the period too of the Dance of Death, of a morbid imagery of decomposing corpses, and of frantic efforts to insure safety and survival after death because the ultimate values human beings still depended on had lost most of their cultural supports. In an effort to reduce anxiety about death, masses for the dead multiplied; so did provision in wills by the living to lessen the dura-tion of their own torment in Purgatory. For the same reason, this was also the period of indulgence mongering—though technically indulgences were never "sold"—that was the immediate occasion of the Protestant revolt, itself the source of further uncertainties. This was a time, too, when the rich and famous constructed ornate tombs for themselves, a kind of sym-bolic protection against the ravages of death.

A vivid representation of these concerns occurred in Florence, that cen-ter of Renaissance magnificence, in 1551, when the Grand Duke sponsored a spectacle for his people on the eve of Lent—a time for repentance. A huge black cart, drawn by black oxen and loaded with human bones and white crosses, carried an enormous figure of Death wielding a sickle. At each place where this vehicle stopped, tomb slabs opened so that those watching could see decomposing cadavers emerging from the graves. Following the cart were persons wearing ghastly death masks, carrying torches, and sing-ing hymns (Gonzalez-Crussi 1994, 79).

Further testimony to this preoccupation with death crops up in unlikely places. Thus Sir Walter Raleigh concluded his *History of the World* with a remarkable tribute to the power of death. "O eloquent, just and mightie Death!" he exclaimed, "Whom none could advise, thou hast persuaded; what none hath dared, thou hast done; and whom all the world hath flattered, thou only hast cast out of the world and despised: thou hast drawne together all the farre stretched greatnesse, all the pride, crueltie and ambition of man, and covered it all over with these two narrow words, *Hic iacet*" (Greenblatt 1973, 153).

Galileo had a rather different experience with the death anxieties of the age. He was under attack from religious conservatives for his new vision of the universe. He saw the cosmos as an infinite space in which the various heavenly bodies could be seen to change position in relation to each other, and thus could no longer supply a spatial location for human beings. The disorientation this occasioned, far more than any scientific objections, was the cause of Galileo's heresy trial. He himself shrewdly recognized why his discoveries aroused so much resistance. His enemies were motivated, he wrote, "by their great desire to go on living, and by the terror they have of death. They do not reflect that if men were immortal, they would never have come into the [changeable] world. Such men really deserve to encounter a Medusa's head which would transmute them into statues of jasper or of diamond, and thus make them more perfect [because immobile and unchanging] than they are."[2] The dread of change and therefore of death that Galileo recognized is still with us.

THE RATIONAL RESPONSE TO DEATH

The central question with which I was concerned as I listened to the other participants in this conference was what, if anything, can be done to alleviate the fear of death that has been so much a part of our own time, as it was during the Renaissance. There is, of course, the rational response to death, of which Galileo was a good example: the view that because it is a function of time and change death should be accepted as a natural and inevitable event. Montaigne, for whom I share Lee Palmer Wandel's affection, sometimes tried to take this view of the matter, which he thought would be the ultimate achievement of philosophy. "To philosophize," he declared in one of his early essays, "is to learn to die" (1967, 56–68).

This was also the view of death taken by that most rational of men, Thomas Jefferson, in a letter to John Adams, quoted with approval by Sherwin Nuland (1994, 73). "There is a ripeness of time for death," Jefferson wrote, "regarding others as well as ourselves, when it is reasonable we should drop off, and make room for another growth. When we have lived our generation out, we should not wish to encroach on another." In this view, then, death can be made relatively familiar and acceptable, and anxiety about it can be kept under control, if not eliminated altogether, through reason. Much that is associated with the literary-ethical tradition of the *ars moriendi* belongs in this school of thought. The genre of the *ars moriendi* isn't so much about death itself as about training the minds of the living to *accept* death, often by so emphasizing the defects in life that death itself, especially the hopeful death of Christians, seems preferable. A grim version of this outlook is represented by Pierre de Bérulle, a French theologian of the early seventeenth century. "The world," Bérulle wrote, "is the scaffold of our execution: we are not only forced to die but condemned to die" (Adam 1959). His contemporary, the Venetian historian Paolo Sarpi, struck a marginally lighter note suggestive of the Mexican Day of the Dead: "Life," he wrote, "is a frivolity to be passed in laughing at death" (1961, 179).

We may well ask then whether this thoroughly rational view of death is a plausible option for human beings in the general absence of that religious hope on which Bérulle and Sarpi depended. In answering this question I think it is helpful to bear in mind that this was the attitude toward death of the ancient Stoics. But even among the Stoics the rational response to death was thought possible only for a tiny minority of sages who had devoted their entire lives to an ascetic and contemplative life in preparation for death. I leave it to you to decide whether Tolstoy's peasants, who may have been wise but were not philosophers, provide a plausible model for the simple acceptance of death. But I note that, according to Boswell, even Dr. Johnson, that most reasonable of men and also a devout Christian, confessed he had "never had a moment in which death was not terrible to him." "No rational man," he declared, "can die without uneasy apprehension" (1933, 2:117, 223, 524). The traditional view of man as a rational animal—itself a cultural artifact much contested in antiquity as well as more recently—seems hardly adequate to reconcile any large proportion of the human race to death. My own suspicion is that rational control over our fears and feelings is the least plausible prescription for reconciliation with death, and that the most desirable—and perhaps difficult—change in our way of dealing with death would be precisely to relinquish the obsession with a control that is, in any case, finally bound to fail. What Jefferson was really describing was not control but submission. And ultimately I find it doubtful whether Stoic indifference can be described as the "reasonable" response to the uncertainty surrounding death.

MAKING DEATH EASIER IN OUR CULTURE

Do the various ways of dealing with death so interestingly discussed in this book, then, suggest ways in which it might be made easier in our culture? I regret that I am not optimistic even in the case of the Western religious traditions, which are increasingly marginalized rather than central to modern culture. Although I have been struck by the frequency with which the words "spiritual" and "spirituality" have figured in the various presentations here, I have had difficulty discerning any clear meaning in this language. I also see little prospect for a religious revival such as has occurred periodically in the Western past. Nor do I find the description of non-Western ways of dealing with death of much use for our purposes. Cultures are something like natural growths. They are not sets of interchangeable parts such that one culture can borrow from another, and they change only very gradually. Little can be done deliberately to change them, although the disintegration of traditional cultures in the modern world suggests that they can be destroyed.

But I do not want to end on so pessimistic a note. For the contributors to this book have from time to time suggested that there may be ways in which our culture is changing for the better—however gradually—in its dealings with death. There is the greater openness to the subject sensed by Ariès, especially among the laity, which suggests that attitudes toward death are becoming (if I may make the distinction) more natural, if not more rational. There is the slight improvement in medical textbooks noted by Joanne Lynn. There are changes in birthing, partly in response to pressures from women. The spread of the hospice movement described by Florence Wald, a development in which she has played so prominent a part, seems particularly promising in its combination of realism and caring. And finally, though I am in no position to generalize about its significance, there has been the conference that led to this book and perhaps others like it elsewhere. I have been profoundly impressed by the concern and sensitivity, the humanity and eloquence, and even the humility of the medical professionals and the other participants in this project—which is itself perhaps a symptom of changing attitudes and a changing culture.

Notes

1. I have dealt with these matters at greater length in "Anxiety and the Formation of Early Modern Culture," included in Bouwsma 1990, 157–89.

2. Galilei 1953, 59. The point here is Galileo's refusal to associate change over time with death, which was the concern of his critics.

References

Adam, A. 1959. *Sur le problème religieux dans la première moitié du XVIIe siècle.* Oxford: Clarendon.

Ariès, P. 1977. *L'homme devant la mort.* Paris: Editions du Seuil.

———. 1981. *The hour of our death.* Trans. Helen Weaver. New York: Knopf.

Boswell, J. 1933. *Life of Samuel Johnson.* Oxford stand. ed. New York: Oxford University Press.

Bouwsma, W. 1990. *A usable past: Essays in European cultural history.* Berkeley: University of California Press.

Galilei, G. 1953. *Dialogue concerning the two chief world systems.* Trans. Stillman Drake. Berkeley: University of California Press.

Gonzalez-Crussi, F. 1993. *The day of the dead and other mortal reflections.* New York: Harcourt Brace.

Greenblatt, S. J. 1973. *Sir Walter Ralegh: The Renaissance man and his roles.* Chicago: University of Chicago Press.

Montaigne, M. (de). 1957. *The complete essays of Montaigne.* Trans. Donald M. Frame. Stanford, Calif.: Stanford University Press.

Nuland, S. B. 1994. *How we die: Reflections on life's final chapter.* New York: Knopf.

Sarpi, P. 1961. *Lettere ai Gallicani* (letter to Giacomo Badoer), 30 March 1609. Ed. Boris Ulianich. Wiesbaden: Franz Steiner Verlag.

ALAN B. ASTROW, M.D., is the acting chief of the section of medical oncology and the program director in hematology and oncology at St. Vincent's Hospital and Medical Center of New York. He is a member of the hospital's ethics committee and has published in the fields of history of medicine and medical ethics. He is a participant in the Wexner Heritage Foundation's program in adult Jewish studies.

WILLIAM J. BOUWSMA, PH.D., is Sather Professor Emeritus of History at the University of California at Berkeley. He was educated at Harvard. He has worked in various areas of European religious and cultural history between the fourteenth and eighteenth centuries and chiefly on French and Italian materials. His major books include: *Venice and the Defense of Republican Liberty* (1968); *John Calvin: A Sixteenth-Century Life* (1988); and *A Usable Past: Essays in European Cultural History* (1990). He has been president of the American Historical Association, the Society for Reformation Research, and the Society for Italian Historical Studies.

DANIEL CALLAHAN, PH.D., is the cofounder and president of The Hastings Center, Briarcliff Manor, New York. For the past twenty-seven years, Callahan has worked in the field of biomedical ethics, with a particular interest in issues of health care rationing and allocation, the way medicine understands mortality, and the relationship of medicine and the broader culture of society. He is the author or editor of thirty-one books, and has written on a variety of issues over his career.

MARY GODENNE MCCREA CURNEN, M.D., DR.P.H., was born in Belgium where she received her M.D. from Louvain University. She came to the United States in 1949 to pursue her career in pediatrics, working in virology at Yale University. After obtaining a Dr.P.H. at Columbia University in 1973, she devoted her research and teaching to cancer epidemiology, which she continued to pursue after returning to Yale in 1982. Her publications have been in virology and cancer epidemiology. She is currently associate director of the Program for Humanities in Medicine at Yale and managing editor of its publications, including *Empathy and the Practice of Medicine* (1993). She is on the editorial board of the *Yale Journal of Biology and Medicine,* which welcomes papers on the humanities.

JOHN DEMOS, PH.D., is Samuel Knight Professor of American History at Yale. His research and writing for many years has focused on social experience in early America. His books include *A Little Commonwealth: Family Life in Plymouth Colony* (1970); *Entertaining Satan: Witchcraft and the Culture of Early New England* (1982); and *The Unredeemed Captive: A Family Story from Early America* (1994).

VALERIE HANSEN, PH.D., is an associate professor in Yale's history department where she teaches both Chinese and Indian history. She is now working on a social history of the Silk Road between India and China. She is the mother of two little girls, Lydia and Claire, and the author of two books: *Changing Gods in Medieval China* (1990) and *Negotiating Daily Life in Traditional China: How Ordinary People Used Contracts* (1995).

PETER S. HAWKINS, PH.D., M.DIV., is professor of religion and literature at the Yale Divinity School and chairman of the Program in Religion and the Arts at Yale's Institute of Sacred Music. With both a Ph.D. in English from Yale and an M.Div. from Union Theological Seminary in New York, Hawkins teaches a wide range of interdisciplinary courses. He has written on American fiction, the literature of Utopia, and Dante. Hawkins began thinking about the NAMES Project AIDS Memorial Quilt in 1990 and has since published three essays on its place in the history of commemoration; he is currently working on a fourth.

ARTHUR E. IMHOF, PH.D., born in Switzerland in 1939, has been a professor of social history and historical demography at the Free University of Berlin since 1975. His main research interests include the increase in life expectancy in Western society during the last four to five centuries and its consequences on the individual, the family, the community, and society. His two most recent publications in this field as contributor and editor include *Lebenserwartungen in Deutschland, Norwegen und Schweden im 19.*

und 20. Jahrhundert (1994); and "Erfüllt leben—in Gelassenheit sterben: Geschichte und Gegenwart" (1994).

JAMES D. KENNEY, M.D., a physician active in the private practice of internal medicine and rheumatology in New Haven, Connecticut, is a clinical professor of medicine at Yale University School of Medicine. Since 1978 he has also served as the associate dean for postgraduate and continuing medical education at the School of Medicine. Kenney is on the editorial board of *The Medical Letter.* Twice yearly he edits and manages *The Medical Letter* / Yale School of Medicine Continuing Medical Education Program, which has completed its sixteenth year and reaches over thirteen thousand physicians.

DIANE M. KOMP, M.D., is a pediatric hematologist-oncologist and professor of pediatrics at Yale University School of Medicine. She is the author of three books about children with cancer and their families that were written for a general audience and published by Zondervan/ [HarperCollins: *A Window to Heaven: When Children See Life in Death* (1992); *A Child Shall Lead Them: Lessons in Hope from Children with Cancer* (1993); and *Hope Springs from Mended Places: Images of Grace in the Shadows of Life* (1994).

ERIC L. KRAKAUER, M.D., PH.D., studied literature at Columbia and philosophy in Berlin, in Freiburg-im-Breisgau where he was a Fulbright Fellow, and at Yale. He received his Ph.D. in philosophy from Yale for a work on Theodor Adorno's philosophical analysis of technology and totalitarianisms. He also received his M.D. from Yale and served his residency in internal medicine at Yale–New Haven Hospital. He is currently a fellow in general internal medicine and medical ethics at Harvard Medical School, studying ways to improve care of critically ill and terminally ill patients.

IRA M. LAPIDUS, PH.D., is professor of history in the Graduate School at the University of California at Berkeley. Since he began his studies at Harvard, he has worked for more than thirty years on Islam and the history of the Middle East, specializing in studies of religion, politics, and community organization. His books include *Middle Eastern Cities: The Later Middle Ages* (1967); *Islamic Movement: Historical Perspectives* (1983); and *A History of Islamic Societies* (1988). Lapidus was for many years chairman of the Center for Middle Eastern Studies at Berkeley, and is a former president of the Middle East Studies Association.

JOANNE LYNN, M.D., M.A., M.S., is director of The Center to Improve Care of the Dying and a professor of health care services and medicine at the George Washington University Medical Center in Washington, D.C. She received her M.D. in 1974 from Boston University and completed her residency in internal medicine at George Washington University. Lynn earned an M.A. in philosophy and social policy in 1982, and an M.S. in clinical evaluative sciences in 1995. She is codirector of SUPPORT, the Study to Understand Prognoses and Preferences for Outcomes and Risks of Treatments, and was assistant director of the President's Commission for the Study of Ethical Problems in Medicine and Biomedical and Behavioral Research.

WILLIAM B. McCULLOUGH, M.D., B.D., is a practicing general surgeon and surgical oncologist in New Haven, Connecticut. He is assistant clinical professor of surgery at Yale University School of Medicine where he teaches medical students and residents the art and craft of surgery. He graduated from Princeton Theological Seminary prior to graduating from Columbia University's College of Physicians and Surgeons. In addition to publications in the professional literature of medicine and surgery, he has written on the subject of death and dying, including chapters in *But Not to Lose* (1969) and *Religion and Bereavement* (1972).

ALAN C. MERMANN, M.D., is clinical professor of pediatrics and chaplain of the Yale School of Medicine. He is an ordained minister in the United Church of Christ. He teaches a seminar for students from five graduate schools on coping with chronic illness and a seminar for medical students on personal and professional issues of the seriously ill and dying patient. He has published articles on spiritual and professional concerns of physicians and the ways in which they cope with stress, the role love plays in the life of the doctor, the work of a chaplain in a medical school, and the varied needs we all have for careful inspection of our personal lives and the values by which we define them.

ALVIN NOVICK, M.D., professor of biology, Yale University, conducts research on the public-policy, ethics, and community-development aspects of HIV disease. He teaches undergraduate and graduate courses in bioethics and in AIDS and society, and is the editor-in-chief of *AIDS and Public Policy Journal*. His recent publications include analysis of some ethical aspects of clinical trials, the difficulties of coalition building in the HIV realm, HIV prevention education, the problems facing children affected by AIDS, and doctor-assisted death.

SHERWIN B. NULAND, M.D., is clinical professor of surgery at the Yale School of Medicine and honorary attending surgeon at the Yale–New Haven Hospital, where he practiced for thirty years before leaving clinical work to devote himself full-time to medical history, medical ethics, and writing. His book *How We Die* won the National Book Award in 1994 and has been published in seventeen languages.

JAMES E. PONET, M.A., an ordained rabbi, works as Jewish chaplain at Yale University and directs the Hillel Foundation there. He teaches throughout the university and leads a monthly physicians' group that addresses current issues confronting women and men in the medical professions.

PETER A. SELWYN, M.D., is director of the AIDS Clinic and associate director of the AIDS Program at Yale–New Haven Hospital. He is also associate professor of medicine, epidemiology, and public health at Yale University School of Medicine. Selwyn has written extensively on AIDS-related clinical and epidemiologic topics, particularly concerning injection drug users, and has been a care provider for HIV-infected patients since the early 1980s. He has a particular interest in working with patients, families, and other care providers on issues raised at the end of life.

HOWARD M. SPIRO, M.D., was born in 1924 in Cambridge, Massachusetts, but was lucky enough in 1955 to move to New Haven, Connecticut, to establish the section of gastroenterology at Yale University School of Medicine. He headed that section until 1982, when he became director of the Program for Humanities in Medicine. Two of his four children are practicing psychiatrists and one is a nurse practitioner. His wife, Marian, who has kept him from too great a degree of pomposity, retired after twenty years as a schoolteacher and is now a carpenter.

FREDERICK J. STREETS, M.Div., M.S.W., C.I.S.W., chaplain at Yale University, served as pastor of Mount Aery Baptist Church, Bridgeport, Connecticut, for approximately seventeen years. There he led the congregation in developing a number of significant programs addressing the mission of the church in an urban context. He is a graduate of Ottawa University (Kansas), Yale University Divinity School, and the Wurzweiler School of Social Work at Yeshiva University. A licensed clinical social worker, Streets is in the Doctor of Social Welfare degree program at Yeshiva University. His research foci are social work and religious values. He has published in the areas of pastoral care, social work, psychiatry, and religion. Streets has been a member of the Yale Divinity School faculty since 1987 and is the first

African-American and Baptist to hold the position of university chaplain. He is also an assistant clinical professor of social work at the Yale Child Study Center.

SYLVIA VATUK, PH.D., is professor of anthropology at the University of Illinois at Chicago. She is a social anthropologist with extensive field re-search experience in India and is the author of numerous scholarly publica-tions on family and kinship relations, women and gender, and social and cultural aspects of aging in that country. As an outgrowth of her research on the family and social roles of the Indian elderly, she has recently begun teaching and writing in the broader area of cross-cultural gerontology. Currently she is engaged in a historical study of a south Indian Muslim family based on documentary and biographical, as well as ethnographic, source materials.

HARALD WAGNER, D.D., is a Roman Catholic priest and theologian. He is a professor of systematic theology (dogmatics) at the University of Mün-ster (Germany). In addition to his academic activities, Wagner is involved in many forms of cooperation between doctors, nurses, and psychologists who deal with problems of medical ethics. His publications include studies on theology, death and dying, and theoretical and practical aspects of working in hospitals and hospices.

FLORENCE S. WALD, M.N., M.S., while dean of Yale's School of Nursing, fostered a curriculum designed to educate graduate students through nurs-ing practice research. Inspired by Cicely Saunders in 1963, Wald left the deanship in 1968 to apply her skills to the support of dying patients and their families, giving them a choice of compassionate palliative care that eases their suffering when aggressive medical care is no longer appropriate. Wald brought an interdisciplinary team together to test the possibilities of giving such care and, with its help, planned the first hospice in the United States, the Connecticut Hospice. Twenty years later, there were more than two thousand hospices and palliative-care institutions around this country. Wald holds honorary degrees from the University of Bridgeport and Mount Holyoke College and, more recently, a doctor of medical sciences degree from Yale University.

LEE PALMER WANDEL, PH.D., is associate professor of history and reli-gious studies at Yale University. Her publications include *Always Among Us: Images of the Poor in Zwingli's Zurich* (1990) and *Voracious Idols and Violent Hands: Iconoclasm in Reformation Zurich, Strasbourg, and Basel*

(1994). Currently she is working on a book on the Eucharist in the sixteenth century. At Yale, she teaches in and has served as director of undergraduate studies for Directed Studies, an interdisciplinary first-year course on the Western tradition from the Greeks to the modern age.

MORRIS A. WESSEL, M.D., practiced pediatrics for forty-two years in New Haven, Connecticut. In 1969 he, along with Florence Wald, Edward Dobihal, chaplain at Yale–New Haven Hospital, and Ira Goldenberg, professor of surgery at Yale Medical School, initiated a study of patients experiencing a terminal illness. The deliberations of this group led to the establishment of the Connecticut Hospice. His participation in these discussions stimulated his interest in bereavement in childhood. In 1993 he received the American Academy of Pediatrics Practitioner Research Award.